Based on the latest research and recommendations from the American Academy of Pediatrics, this essential handbook answers common questions parents have about attention deficit/ hyperactivity disorder (ADHD), including

- How is ADHD defined today?

- How can I tell if my child's problems are due to ADHD and not some other problem?

- What is the best way to work with my child's teacher?

- What types of medications are used to treat ADHD?

- What steps can I take to help my parenting be as successful as possible?

- Should I involve my child in the treatment plan?

- Are there classroom structures and school policies that will best support my child?

- How can I help my teenager manage social and emotional pressures?

- Can I trust the information available on the Internet?

…and much more, to help improve the quality of life for your child and your family.

Additional Parenting Books From the American Academy of Pediatrics

Common Conditions

ADHD: What Every Parent Needs to Know

Allergies and Asthma: What Every Parent Needs to Know

Waking Up Dry: A Guide to Help Children Overcome Bedwetting

Developmental, Behavioral, and Psychosocial Information

CyberSafe: Protecting and Empowering Kids in the Digital World of Texting, Gaming, and Social Media

Mental Health, Naturally: The Family Guide to Holistic Care for a Healthy Mind and Body

The Wonder Years: Helping Your Baby and Young Child Successfully Negotiate the Major Developmental Milestones

Immunization Information

Immunizations & Infectious Diseases: An Informed Parent's Guide

Newborns, Infants, and Toddlers

Baby & Child Health: The Essential Guide From Birth to 11 Years

Caring for Your Baby and Young Child: Birth to Age 5*

Guide to Toilet Training*

Heading Home With Your Newborn: From Birth to Reality

Mommy Calls: Dr. Tanya Answers Parents' Top 101 Questions About Babies and Toddlers

New Mother's Guide to Breastfeeding*

Newborn Intensive Care: What Every Parent Needs to Know

Raising Twins: From Pregnancy to Preschool Your Baby's First Year*

Nutrition and Fitness

Food Fights: Winning the Nutritional Challenges of Parenthood Armed With Insight, Humor, and a Bottle of Ketchup

A Parent's Guide to Childhood Obesity: A Road Map to Health

Sports Success Rx! Your Child's Prescription for the Best Experience

School-aged Children and Adolescents

Building Resilience in Children and Teens: Giving Kids Roots and Wings

Caring for Your School-Age Child: Ages 5 to 12

Caring for Your Teenager

Less Stress, More Success: A New Approach to Guiding Your Teen Through College Admissions and Beyond

For more information, please visit the official AAP Web site for parents, www.HealthyChildren.org/bookstore.

*This book is also available in Spanish.

ADHD

2ND EDITION

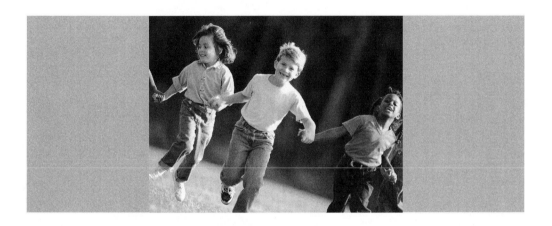

What Every Parent Needs to Know

MICHAEL I. REIFF, MD, FAAP

EDITOR IN CHIEF

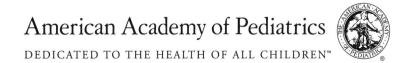

American Academy of Pediatrics

DEDICATED TO THE HEALTH OF ALL CHILDREN™

American Academy of Pediatrics Department of Marketing and Publications Staff

Director, Department of Marketing and Publications
Maureen DeRosa, MPA

Director, Division of Product Development
Mark Grimes

Manager, Consumer Publishing
Carolyn Kolbaba

Manager, Product Development
Eileen Glasstetter, MS

Coordinator, Product Development
Holly Kaminski

Editorial Assistant, Product Development
Carrie Peters

Director, Division of Publishing and Production Services
Sandi King, MS

Manager, Editorial Services
Kate Larson

Print Production Specialist
Shannan Martin

Manager, Art Direction and Production
Linda Diamond

Director, Division of Marketing and Sales
Kevin Tuley

Manager, Consumer Product Marketing
Kathleen Juhl, MBA

Published by the American Academy of Pediatrics
141 Northwest Point Blvd, Elk Grove Village, IL 60007-1019
847/434-4000
Fax: 847/434-8000
www.aap.org

Cover design by Daniel Rembert
Book design by Linda Diamond
Illustrations by Anthony Alex LeTourneau

Second Edition—2011
First Edition—© 2000 as *ADHD: A Complete and Authoritative Guide*

Library of Congress Control Number: 2010943007
ISBN: 978-1-58110-451-6

CB0062
9-167

1 2 3 4 5 6 7 8 9 10

Reviewers/Contributors

Editor in Chief
Michael I. Reiff, MD, FAAP
Associate Professor of Pediatrics
  and Family Medicine
Director, Autism Spectrum and
  Neurodevelopmental Disorders Clinic
Director, Minnesota LEND Program
University of Minnesota
Minneapolis, MN

American Academy of Pediatrics
Board of Directors Reviewer
Michael V. Severson, MD, FAAP

Reviewers and Contributors
Clinical Practice Guideline Subcommittee
on Attention-Deficit/Hyperactivity
Disorder Members
Mark L. Wolraich, MD, FAAP, Chairperson
  (Developmental and Behavioral Pediatrics)
Lawrence W. Brown, MD, FAAP
  (Neurology)
Marian F. Earls, MD, FAAP
  (General Pediatrics, QuIIN)
James M. Perrin, MD, FAAP
  (General Pediatrics, Children With
  Disabilities)
Bruce P. Meyer, MD, FAAP
  (General Pediatrics)
Michael I. Reiff, MD, FAAP
  (Developmental and Behavioral Pediatrics)
Esther Janowsky, MD, PhD
  (Epidemiology, Internal Medicine)

Martin T. Stein, MD, FAAP
  (Developmental and Behavioral Pediatrics)
Susanna N. Visser, MS
  (Epidemiology)

Liaisons/Consultants
Ronald T. Brown, PhD, ABPP
  (American Psychological Association)
George J. DuPaul, PhD
  (National Association of School
  Psychologists)
Heidi M. Feldman, MD, PhD, FAAP
  (Society for Developmental and
  Behavioral Pediatrics)
Theodore G. Ganiats, MD
  (American Academy of Family Physicians)
Beth A. Kaplanek, RN, BSN
  (Children and Adults With Attention-
  Deficit/Hyperactivity Disorder)
Karen L. Pierce, MD
  (American Academy of Child and
  Adolescent Psychiatry)

Medical Writer
Melissa Caper, MA, MFA

Staff
Caryn Davidson, MA

Additional Reviewers and Contributors

Howard Abikoff, PhD

Robert W. Amler, MD, MS, FAAP

Carolyn Anderson

Edward R. Christophersen, PhD, FAAP

Jane M. Foy, MD, FAAP

Harlan R. Gephart, MD, FAAP

Paula F. Goldberg

Ross Greene, PhD

Joseph F. Hagan Jr, MD, FAAP

Julie Holmquist

Charles J. Homer, MD, MPH, FAAP

Kelly J. Kelleher, MD, MPH, FAAP

Christopher J. Kratochvil, MD

Carole M. Lannon, MD, MPH, FAAP

Karen J. Miller, MD, FAAP

Kathleen G. Nadeau, PhD

William E. Pelham Jr, PhD

Patricia O. Quinn, MD, FAAP

Sandra F. Rief, MA

E. Clarke Ross, DPA

Francis E. Rushton Jr, MD, FAAP

Jerry L. Rushton, MD, MPH, FAAP

Howard H. Schubiner, MD, FAAP

Thomas J. Sullivan, MD, FAAP

James Swanson, PhD

Writers

Richard Trubo

Sherill Tippins

Dedication

Listen to the Mustn'ts, child, listen to the Don'ts

Listen to the Shouldn'ts, the Impossibles, the Won'ts.

Listen to the Never Haves, then listen close to me.

Anything can happen, Anything can be

—Shel Silverstein

To Dylan and Jess who have taught me about the rich journey through childhood and adolescence, and young adulthood.

And to all the children, adolescents, young adults and their families who struggle daily to turn the Don'ts and Won'ts of ADHD into the Anything Can Bes.

Table of Contents

Please Note

The information contained in this book is intended to complement, not substitute for, the advice of your child's pediatrician. Before starting any medical treatment or medical program, you should consult with your child's pediatrician, who can discuss your child's individual needs and counsel you about symptoms and treatment. If you have any questions regarding how the information in this book applies to your child, speak to your child's pediatrician.

Foreword

The American Academy of Pediatrics (AAP) welcomes you to the second edition of its popular parenting book, *ADHD: What Every Parent Needs to Know.*

This book will help readers apply the most current evidence-based and best-practice approaches for finding solutions for children with attention-deficit/hyperactivity disorder (ADHD). Many important topics are addressed in this book, including the diagnostic process, behavior therapy, medication, and advice on management techniques for school and home. We encourage its use in concert with the advice and counsel of our readers' pediatricians and hope that it serves to strengthen collaboration among parents, children, primary care professionals, and school personnel.

What separates *ADHD: What Every Parent Needs to Know* from other reference books on this topic is that pediatricians who specialize in this have extensively reviewed it. Under the direction of our editor in chief, the material in this book was developed with the assistance of numerous contributors from the AAP.

The AAP is an organization of 60,000 primary care pediatricians, pediatric medical subspecialists, and pediatric surgical specialists dedicated to the health, safety, and well being of infants, children, adolescents, and young adults. *ADHD: What Every Parent Needs to Know* is part of ongoing AAP educational efforts to provide parents and caregivers with high-quality information on a broad spectrum of children's health issues.

Errol R. Alden, MD, FAAP
Executive Director/CEO
American Academy of Pediatrics

A Note on Gender

A good deal of discussion went into the use of pronouns ("hes" and "shes") for this book, particularly when describing different subtypes of attention-deficit/hyperactivity disorder (ADHD) or different problems faced by children with ADHD. Although boys and girls can have any subtype of ADHD or any of the related problems, the number of boys diagnosed with ADHD is about 3 to 1 over girls, and the combined type of ADHD with all 3 key elements—impulsivity, hyperactivity, and inattention—is diagnosed about 2½ times more frequently than the predominantly inattentive type. However, if all the children in a school system were evaluated, it is likely that the inattentive type would be found to be about 1½ times more common than the combined type—this inattentive type is just more likely to go undiagnosed, and girls are more likely to have this subtype than boys. With this as background, we have attempted to balance the "hes" and "shes" in this book in an interchangeable way.

Introduction

Why Another Book About ADHD?

Almost all children have times when their attention or behavior veers out of control. However, for some children, these types of behaviors are more than an occasional problem. Children with attention deficit/hyperactivity disorder (ADHD) have behavior problems that are so frequent and significant that they interfere with their ability to function adequately on a daily basis. Attention-deficit/hyperactivity disorder is the most commonly diagnosed developmental-behavioral condition in children, affecting approximately 6% to 9% of the school-aged population. It is a chronic condition whose symptoms continue in 60% to 80% of adolescents and, in some individuals, even into adulthood. It can have effects on children's learning, ability to regulate their behavior, social skills, and self esteem.

Attention-deficit/hyperactivity disorder is the most researched of all childhood behavioral disorders, with more than 1,000 scientific articles published yearly. Yet a great deal of controversy still exists in the media and in the general public about the nature of ADHD and the best means of treatment. You are probably already aware of the variety of books on ADHD dominating the "parenting" shelves of your local bookstore. Web sites also abound with an enormous amount of information for parents, ranging from carefully researched to highly irresponsible. This glut of advice can be mind-boggling for parents to sort out. Attention-deficit/hyperactivity disorder is reported by the media to be overdiagnosed and underdiagnosed, and overtreated and undertreated all at the same time. Descriptions of the same new medication can range from "groundbreaking" to "dangerous." How can a responsible parent sort through this quagmire of seemingly contradictory data? A major goal of this book is helping parents to answer this question: Why all the confusion? If only ADHD was as easy to diagnose as, say, diabetes or asthma. But unfortunately, as you will learn in chapters 1 and 2, there is no laboratory test for ADHD, no urine or blood test, x-ray, or brain wave study that can tell you definitively whether your child has ADHD. Instead, your child's treatment team consisting of you, your child, his medical team, teachers, and others who know and work with him—will work together to analyze your child's *functioning*—that is, whether and how his symptoms seriously affect his behavior, learning, social skills, and/or self esteem at home, at school, or in other situations. This is done through careful observation, exchange of information, the completion of behavior-rating questionnaires, and other steps as outlined in the latest research based guidelines developed by the American Academy of Pediatrics that you will read about in chapters 1 and 2. The diagnostic process can be complicated by the fact that some other conditions, such as anxiety or depression and behavior disorders, can seem quite similar to ADHD and often accompany, or "coexist with" the condition. These will be reviewed in detail in Chapter 9. With this information in hand, it is certainly possible to accurately diagnose ADHD in a way that can lead to effective treatment.

What do we know about treatment? Physicians and psychologists are constantly juggling and integrating several levels of information in their attempt to help you and your family find the best solutions and outcomes for your child with ADHD. The most reliable and consistent information is what we call evidence-based. Evidence-based medicine unites the unique clinical expertise of your child's physician with the best clinical evidence from systematic research studies in making decisions about the care of your child and family. In chapters 3 through 7 you will learn that the only 2 treatments for ADHD that are strongly evidence-based are medication and behavior therapy. The good news is that these treatments have been found to be effective in rigorous clinical studies. The challenge is that some of the procedures and routines used in these clinical studies are not easily available in real life situations. This is why it is so important to work with your own child's clinicians and educators to adapt as many of the principles of "ideal management" described in this book to your own family circumstances and to the unique needs of your child. Although monthly visits for medication management may be ideal (but not practical), for example, you and your child's pediatrician may decide that many of the same goals can be accomplished by carefully planned visits every 3 to 4 months. Likewise, the type of systematic parent training described in Chapter 6 may not be readily available in your community, or may not be covered by your insurance plan. Still, you can adapt many of these principles after reading the chapter, and may find it even more useful to work with a child therapist to modify these techniques even if it is not in the exact systematic approach described here. The types of summer school and camp programs described in Chapter 7 also may not be readily available in your community, but their principles can be adapted to many classroom and other group situations. These programs also can be used as models by parents when advocating for needed community services that have been proven effective.

In some cases, especially with ADHD and related disorders, not enough studies have been done to indicate an effective, evidence-based approach to a given problem, even though the need for help is clear. In these cases, a best practice approach is the best alternative. A best practice approach is based on a consensus of what experts consider the best advice in the absence of definitive studies. Many of the suggestions in chapters 5, 7, 11, and 12, especially those on effective management techniques for home and school in addition to behavior therapy, are based on this best practice approach.

If sorting out the material for parents written by recognized experts (some of these are included as recommendations in the Resources section on page 311) is difficult, knowing what to make of other books, material from Web sites, information from parent chat rooms, etc, can be daunting. Some of the more controversial, unproven, and alternative treatments proposed for ADHD are reviewed in Chapter 10. Consumer beware! Some of these treatments, like eliminating sugar from the diet, have been shown to be ineffective. Others, such as biofeedback, are time consuming and costly, and have not been studied systematically enough to be able to recommend them. In Chapter 10 you will find information on how to judge claims of treatment success by analyzing the evidence and considering the source of the information, whether there is a scientific basis for the claim, and whether an unstated motive (such as making a sale) may underlie claims for a particular theory or treatment plan. Your child's pediatrician can be an excellent resource in helping to evaluate ADHD-related information and likely has had experience with many families who have applied a wide spectrum of approaches to help their children with ADHD.

This book strongly recommends that you consider evidence-based or best practice approaches as the mainstay of any evaluation or treatment plan, and that alternative treatments be tried only after a critical discussion with the professionals on your child's treatment team. So read this book and any other materials on ADHD diagnosis, evaluation, or treatment critically! Always ask yourself if the material presented is evidence-based or reflects best practice, sound expert advice, someone's belief based only on what they did for their own child, an opinion criticizing established treatments for some political agenda, an attempt to sell an unproven product, etc, and draw your own informed conclusions.

Finally, will following the advice in this book lead to a better long-term result for your child and your family? Surprisingly, the number of long-term studies are extremely limited especially those using the types of evidence based approaches to treatment that we recommend. Such studies are costly, require large numbers of families, and can be difficult to interpret because of all the ways that real life considerations impose themselves on individual children in different ways over a long study period. In addition, as you will read in this book, the last few years have led to major advances in our knowledge about ADHD, and it will take several years to be able to see how these advances translate into better outcomes over a long period. Having said that, we remain optimistic that by using the information contained in this book, you will be applying the most current evidence based and best practice approaches for improving the life and functioning of your child.

Chapter 1

What Is ADHD?

Andrew Scott had always been an active child. From the time he learned to walk his parents noticed he was "into everything." Andrew's preschool teachers frequently commented on how active he was, and his kindergarten teacher observed that he was "quite a handful." First grade passed without any major problems, though his level of activity seemed to overwhelm some of the other children during playtime. In third grade, however, Andrew began to fall behind in math and reading. His teacher said he was too restless. During class he bothered the children around him. He seemed unable to focus on a learning activity for longer than a few minutes. On the playground he was "over-physical" with his peers, invading their space and then overreacting when they pushed him away.

Around the middle of the year, Andrew's teacher met with his parents. She told them that she believed Andrew's problems paying attention, his high activity level, and troubles with schoolwork might indicate the presence of attention-deficit/hyperactivity disorder (ADHD). She explained that ADHD often goes undetected until children enter school and academics and social relationships begin to be affected.

Despite the teacher's positive attitude, Andrew's parents were stunned by her recommendation that their son be evaluated for ADHD. They had always been challenged by their active child, but they had never considered his behavior out of the ordinary for a healthy young boy. As Andrew's father often pointed out, Andrew was "just like me when I was in school"—eager, excited, and always on the go. While both parents agreed that Andrew could use some extra help with his social skills and reading, they did not see how these behaviors could be thought of as a medical condition. "I think his teacher just can't handle him in class," Andrew's mother told her husband later when they were back at home. "She has a discipline problem and she calls it ADHD. I think it's the school that should be evaluated."

The Keller family was experiencing similar confusion. Their 12-year-old daughter, Emma, was also having problems. However, she was on the quiet and somewhat anxious side. Since early childhood, she had been a "dreamer" whose thoughts tended to drift easily. She often forgot things she had recently learned or been told, and spent much of her time alone. In recent years, her "randomness" and lack of organization had begun to seriously affect her school performance, social life, and family relationships. She was having trouble completing tasks and was messy and careless about her schoolwork. Her parents noted that she was often forgetful and at times it seemed as if her mind was elsewhere and that she was not listening. Still, Emma's parents felt that her behavior was typical of many girls her age and was nothing that a little maturation and help with organization could not cure. Was it really necessary, they asked Emma's pediatrician, to consider this a medical issue or to start an evaluation for ADHD as he had suggested?

As different as Andrew's and Emma's situations seem to be, both are typical for children with ADHD. Attention-deficit/hyperactivity disorder limits children's ability to filter out irrelevant input, focus, organize, prioritize, delay gratification, think before they act, or perform other so-called executive functions that most of us perform automatically. In children such as Andrew, with "hyperactive-impulsive" elements to his ADHD, the disorder presents itself as an inability to control impulses or regulate activity levels, even when the child knows how he is expected to behave. In those with "inattentive-type" ADHD, including Emma, an inability to filter information means that someone walking by the classroom can claim as much attention as the teacher's lecture, and that a date with a friend can be forgotten in a flood of unregulated input.

Because these behaviors—short attention span, forgetfulness, inability to sit still, unusually high activity level, and a tendency to act before thinking—are also common in children with and without ADHD, many families are surprised when their child is referred for an evaluation. Adding to their confusion is the fact that all of these behaviors occur in children and adolescents throughout their development, although those with ADHD exhibit more extreme and immature forms of these behaviors. These behaviors interfere in significant ways with their day-to-day functioning, and they do not outgrow them at the same pace that other children do. Because other disorders, such as learning disabilities, oppositional defiant disorder, and anxiety or depression, can resemble ADHD (and, in fact, often accompany it), it can be difficult to tell whether a child has another condition, ADHD, or both. Finally, the fact that ADHD is diagnosed through careful observations of inattentive, hyperactive, and impulsive behaviors across the major settings of a child's life—rather than the types of laboratory procedures used to diagnose such disorders as diabetes—leads some adults and the popular press to question whether ADHD exists at all.

Yet a large body of convincing evidence suggests that ADHD is a biological, brain-based condition. The scientific research on ADHD is more thorough and compelling than for most behavioral and mental health disorders, and even many medical conditions. Even so, among many parents it remains controversial and misunderstood. In 1998 the National Institutes of Health, responding to public concern and debate about ADHD diagnosis and treatment, assembled a group of experts for a consensus conference on ADHD. These experts published their conclusions stating that ADHD is indeed a medical disorder.

According to recent estimates, ADHD is among the most prevalent chronic childhood disorders, occurring in 6% to 9% of school-aged children (second only to asthma). The Centers for Disease Control and Prevention has reported that about 4.5 million children (ages 3–17) in the United States have ADHD, and the condition currently accounts for as many as 30% to 50% of child referrals to mental health services. Many people believe that the prevalence of ADHD has increased significantly in recent decades, perhaps due to environmental factors, but there is no convincing evidence that this is the case. The number of children who have ADHD has likely remained roughly stable, but the number of children diagnosed with the condition has increased as more clinicians have become familiar with its symptoms and the criteria for diagnosing ADHD have changed.

A generally reliable method for diagnosing ADHD based on the child's behavior and functioning has been established. Parents whose children have been adequately evaluated for ADHD, and who have implemented appropriate treatment as a result, frequently report that the difference before and after their child's treatment is "like night and day." While ADHD cannot be cured, children can be helped to compensate for their problems so that school performance and social relationships improve. As a result, their self-esteem increases, as do their chances for future successes.

In this book, you will learn how ADHD is defined and recognized; how it is evaluated; and how, according to the latest reliable scientific research, it can best be treated. Researchers have identified the types of behavioral, academic, and social supports most likely to be useful at school and at home, and courses and therapies have been developed to pass this information on to parents and teachers in the community. You will also learn about special concerns in the evaluation and treatment of preschoolers and adolescents with ADHD, and the changing effect of this chronic condition over time. This is not to say that we now know everything there is to know about the nature and proper treatment of ADHD. A number of questions remain to be answered, and there is a great deal of research still to be done. Active, ongoing studies may provide further insight into how your child can improve his experience at each stage of life. The good news is that the evaluation and treatment of ADHD is at a much more advanced stage today than ever before. Armed with the knowledge provided to you in these pages, you and your child will be able to address the challenges of ADHD with confidence and optimism.

Before learning about how ADHD is recognized, diagnosed, and treated, however, it is necessary to understand exactly what ADHD is—and what it is not. In this chapter you will learn

- How the view of ADHD has evolved over time
- How ADHD is defined today
- What scientists believe may cause ADHD
- How the condition typically alters a child's experience and what its long-term effects are

Through it all, always keep in mind that you have "a child with ADHD," rather than "an ADHD child." He is a child first and foremost, and the problems associated with ADHD can be worked on. Never lose sight of the whole picture.

MYTHS AND MISCONCEPTIONS ABOUT ADHD

Much misinformation has circulated about ADHD and its causes, diagnosis, and treatment over recent decades. Following are a number of untrue assumptions about the disorder, along with explanations aimed at clarifying the issues.

- **"My preschooler is too young to have ADHD."** Many parents believe that ADHD is a problem of school-aged children. But, in fact, the symptoms of ADHD, and the diagnosis of the condition, can occur as early as the preschool years. At times, even doctors have difficulty differentiating "normal" behavior from those suggesting ADHD in a preschooler. Although a young child may normally have characteristics like impulsive or hyperactive behavior, these can be symptoms of ADHD as well. A pediatrician will evaluate the intensity of these behaviors in a preschooler to help in making the diagnosis. Attention-deficit/hyperactivity disorder is diagnosed when these problems get to the point where they are significantly and consistently interfering with a preschooler's life, development, self-esteem and general functioning.

- **"He's just lazy and unmotivated."** This assumption is a common response to the behavior exhibited by a child who is struggling with ADHD. A child who finds it nearly impossible to stay focused in class, or to complete a lengthy task such as writing a long essay, may try to save face by acting as though he does not want to do it or is too lazy to finish. This behavior may look like laziness or lack of motivation, but it stems from real difficulty in functioning. All children want to succeed and get praised for their good work. If such tasks were easy for children with ADHD to accomplish, and provided rewarding feedback, those children would seem just as "motivated" as anyone else.

- **"He's a handful—or, she's a daydreamer—but that's normal. They just don't let kids be kids these days."** It is true that all children are impulsive, active, and inattentive at times, sometimes to the extreme. A child with ADHD, however, is more than just a "handful" for his parents and teachers, or a "daydreamer" who tends to lose herself in thought. His or her hyperactivity and/or inattentiveness constitute a real day-to-day functional disability. That is, it seriously and consistently impedes the ability to succeed at school, fit into family routines, follow household rules, maintain friendships, interact positively with family members, avoid injury, or otherwise manage in his or her environment. As you will learn in Chapter 2, this clear functional disability is what pediatricians look for when diagnosing ADHD and recommending treatment.

MYTHS AND MISCONCEPTIONS ABOUT ADHD (CONTINUED)

- **"Treatment for ADHD will cure it. The goal is to get off medication as soon as possible."** Attention-deficit/hyperactivity disorder is a chronic condition that often does not entirely go away, but instead changes form over time. Many older adolescents and adults are able to organize their lives and use techniques that allow them to forego medical treatment, although a significant number continue various forms of treatment and support throughout their life spans. Depending on the circumstances and demands as a person matures, this may or may not include continuing with medication or other treatments for ADHD at different times, even through adult life. The true goal is to function well at each stage of childhood and adolescence, and as an adult, rather than to stop any or all treatments as soon as possible.

- **"He focuses on his video games for hours. He can't have ADHD."** For the most part ADHD poses problems with tasks that require focused attention over long periods, not so much for activities that are highly engaging or stimulating. School can be especially challenging for a person with ADHD because the typical classroom lecture, compared with a video game, can be relatively unstimulating in terms of visuals, sound, and physical activity. Assignments can be long and require sustained, organized thought and effort, and the daily routine can be less structured and predictable than a child with ADHD might require. Most children with ADHD are diagnosed during their school years precisely because the academic, social, and behavioral demands during these years are so difficult for them. The difficulties that such children experience may make it seem that school is the problem (and, certainly, that possibility should be considered), but it is more likely to be a result of the child's struggle to manage in this environment.

  Other situations that can be problematic for children with ADHD include social interactions, with their constant, subtle exchange of emotional and social information; sports that require a high degree of focus or concentration; and extracurricular activities that require them to sit still, listen, or wait their turn for long periods.

- **"ADHD is caused by poor parental discipline."** Attention-deficit/hyperactivity disorder is not a result of poor discipline—although behaviors that stem from ADHD can challenge otherwise effective parenting styles. Inconsistent limit-setting and other ineffective parenting practices can, however, worsen its expression. In chapters 5 and 6 you will find a number of proven parenting techniques that can help children with ADHD manage their behavior.

MYTHS AND MISCONCEPTIONS ABOUT ADHD (CONTINUED)

- **"If, after a careful evaluation, a child doesn't receive the ADHD diagnosis, she doesn't need help."** Attention-deficit/hyperactivity disorder is diagnosed on a continuum, which means that a child can exhibit a number of ADHD-type behaviors yet not to the extent that she is diagnosed with ADHD. This does not mean she needs no help coping with the problems that she does have. The family of a child who does not meet the criteria for ADHD but has similar problems may be offered pediatric counseling, education about the range of normal developmental behaviors, home behavior management tools, school behavior management recommendations, social skills interventions, and help with managing homework flow and with organization and planning.

- **"Children with ADHD outgrow this condition."** Parents and many doctors once believed that as children with ADHD enter adolescence and then move into adulthood, their ADHD will no longer be an issue. But recent studies have shown that some aspects of ADHD can persist well into adult life for as many as 85% of these children. Some adults can still benefit from the use of ADHD medication for the rest of their lives. Others have demonstrated enough improvement that this medication becomes unneeded depending on what occupation they choose and their ability to succeed in relationships and other social activities. No matter what the circumstances of particular adults may be, however, they can make adjustments in their environment, take full advantage of their own strengths, and lead very productive adult lives, even when aspects of ADHD still persist.

How Is ADHD Defined?

On television, in magazines and newspapers, and in thousands of everyday conversations, there is ongoing debate around whether certain "ADHD-type" behaviors lie within the realm of normal childhood experience or constitute a disorder that requires treatment. The issue of exactly where and how to draw the line between typical behavior and a clinical condition may become even clearer as increasingly sophisticated diagnostic techniques provide researchers with more information about the nature of the precise brain processes involved in children with ADHD, but the use of these tools and techniques for these purposes still lies in the future.

For more than a century physicians have been aware of children displaying the behaviors that we now call ADHD. In 1902 British pediatrician George Still first formally documented a condition in which children seemed inattentive, impulsive, and hyperactive, stating his belief that this was a result of biological makeup rather than poor parenting or other environmental factors. Research in the 1980s supported this hypothesis and led to the use of the term *attention deficit disorder.* In 1987, in response to even more precise information provided by new studies, the term *attention-deficit/hyperactivity disorder* was introduced.

Today ADHD is defined by the American Psychiatric Association as developmentally inappropriate attention and/or hyperactivity and impulsivity so pervasive and persistent as to significantly interfere with a child's daily life. A child with ADHD has difficulty controlling his behavior in most major settings, including home and school. He may speed about in constant motion, make noise nonstop, refuse to wait his turn, and crash into everything around him. At other times he may drift as if in a daydream, failing to pay attention to or

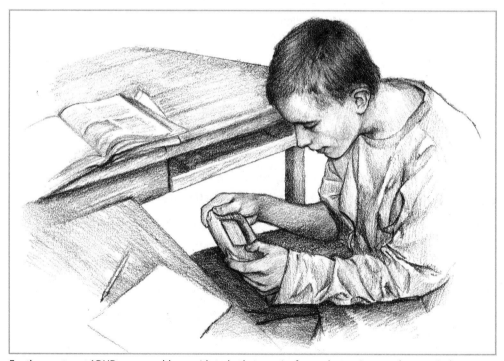

For the most part ADHD poses problems with tasks that require focused attention over long periods, not so much for activities that are highly engaging or stimulating, such as a video game.

finish what he starts. He may have trouble learning and remembering. An impulsive nature may put him in actual physical danger. Because he has difficulty controlling this behavior, he may be labeled a "bad kid" or a "space cadet." These problems begin to occur relatively early in life (before age 7 years), though they sometimes go unrecognized until later. However, if there are absolutely no indications of ADHD before age 7 years, an alternative explanation for a child's later behaviors should be sought.

Professionals have identified clear differences between the functioning of a child without ADHD and a child with the condition. The presence of ADHD may be suspected if the

1. Inattentive, impulsive, or hyperactive behavior is not age-appropriate. That is, if it is not typical of children of the same age who do not have ADHD.
2. Behavior leads to chronic problems in daily functioning. A mild tendency to daydream or an active temperament, which may cause occasional problems for a child but is not seriously disabling, is not considered evidence of ADHD.
3. Behavior is natural to the child and not a result of poor care, physical injury, abuse or neglect, disease, or other environmental influence. One way to determine whether the problem is environmental is to look at whether the problem occurs in more than one setting, such as at home and at school. If not, then an environmental cause, such as stresses at home or an inappropriate classroom placement, is more likely than ADHD to be the cause of the problem for the child.

For a child's condition to be diagnosed as ADHD, *all* 3 of these conditions must be met. Attention-deficit/hyperactivity disorder can only be recognized by its symptoms, and by the problems that these symptoms create for the child. This is why it is so important for parents, teachers, mental health professionals, and medical experts to work together when evaluating a child for ADHD. Each contributes his or her own observations, experience, and expertise to create a comprehensive picture of the child's social, academic, and emotional progress.

Attention-deficit/hyperactivity disorder is divided into 3 general subtypes: *predominantly hyperactive-impulsive–type ADHD, predominantly inattentive-type ADHD,* and *combined-type ADHD.* A child with predominantly hyperactive-impulsive–type ADHD may fidget or squirm in his seat, have difficulty waiting his turn, and show a tendency to be disorganized.

He may act immaturely, have a poor sense of physical boundaries, and tend toward destructive behaviors and conduct problems. A child with predominantly inattentive-type ADHD, on the other hand, may seem distracted and "spacey" or "daydreamy," but lacks the hyperactive component of the disorder. He may seem to process information slowly and may also have a learning disorder, anxiety, or depression. A child with combined-type ADHD typically exhibits many of the behaviors of the first 2 subtypes.

GIRLS AND ADHD

The fact that many more boys than girls are diagnosed with ADHD—at a ratio of approximately 2 to 1 or 3 to 1—has led to the mistaken belief among many parents and teachers that ADHD is a "boys' disorder" that rarely occurs in girls. In fact, more girls than boys qualify for the diagnosis of ADHD, but more girls remain undiagnosed because they have the inattentive type of ADHD, and tend to be overlooked entirely or do not attract attention until they are older. This means that girls are less likely to be referred for evaluation and to receive the help they need. Even when diagnosis and treatment have been obtained, girls with ADHD are further disadvantaged by the fact that most ADHD research to date has focused on boys. Little is known about potential differences between the genders in the development of the condition over time or response to medication and other forms of treatment. Compared with other girls, girls with ADHD experience more depression, anxiety, distress, poor teacher relationships, stress, external locus of control (the feeling that "the winds of fate" control their destiny instead of themselves), and impaired academics. Compared with boys with ADHD, girls with ADHD experience more difficulties from feeling anxious, distressed, or depressed, and less of a feeling that they can take control in solving problems that they face.

If your daughter has been referred for evaluation for ADHD, or if you suspect that she may have the condition, it is important not to discount the possibility just because she is female. Teachers tend to under-refer girls for evaluation, even when their symptoms are the same as boys', and girls are less likely than boys to receive sufficient medical treatment once they have been diagnosed. Be aware that some sociocultural beliefs about girls (that they tend to daydream, that they just are not interested in academics) may mask a real problem in your child's ability to function. If your daughter is diagnosed with ADHD, ask the pediatrician to keep you updated on ongoing research about the development of ADHD in girls, the particular challenges girls with ADHD are likely to meet, and the different ways in which they may respond to various forms of treatment.

These subtypes tend to be diagnosed at different ages and stages of development. Because of the hyperactivity and impulsivity, children with predominantly hyperactive-impulsive type or combined type may be diagnosed as early as the preschool years in extreme situations. Children with predominantly inattentive type often go undetected until fourth grade or even later, when increased demands for sustained attention and more homework lead to significant problems in functioning. In the early grades children learn to read, but at around fourth grade they need to begin to read to learn. When this transition takes place, children with inattentive type typically begin to have more problems.

While the problems of hyperactivity/impulsivity and inattentiveness may seem at first to be unrelated, they both influence a child's inability to focus and function well in school, with peers, and in the family. Attention-deficit/hyperactivity disorder can be thought of as a range of "attentional disorders" with a number of possible symptoms shown at different ages and developmental stages.

What Causes ADHD?

No single cause has yet been identified for ADHD. A number of risk factors have been noted, however, that affect a child's brain development and behavior that acting in combination may lead to ADHD symptoms. They include genetic factors, variations in temperament (a child's individual differences in emotional reactivity, activity level, attention, and self-regulation), medical causes (especially those that affect brain development), and a host of environmental influences on the developing brain (including toxins such as lead, alcohol, and nutritional deficiencies). Some research finds that children with ADHD may experience a delay in the normal maturing of their brain. Despite these many advances in research on the causes of ADHD, none of these findings are yet ready for use by physicians in making the diagnosis of ADHD.

Researchers are certain that ADHD tends to run in families. Close relatives of people with ADHD have about a 5 times greater than random chance of having ADHD themselves, as well as a higher risk for such common accompanying disorders as anxiety, depression, learning disabilities, and conduct disorders. An identical twin is at high risk of sharing his twin's ADHD, and a sibling of a child with ADHD has about a 30% chance of having similar problems. Although no single gene has been identified for ADHD, research continues in this area, and it is likely that several genes will be found that contribute to ADHD symptoms. Brain imaging studies have found some differences in brain anatomy between children diagnosed with ADHD and those who have not been diagnosed, but no consistent pattern has yet emerged from these studies. The fact that children and adolescents respond so consistently to stimulant medications, and that these medications influence biochemical systems in the brain, suggests that biochemical causes may contribute to ADHD symptoms as well. This remains an area of active research. In the next few years newer brain-imaging tools and more sophisticated genetic techniques will continue to shed more light on the processes underlying ADHD. Still, it is unlikely that a single cause will be identified.

ADHD Over Time

Attention-deficit/hyperactivity disorder is a complex disorder with different challenges arising at each new phase of a child's development. Children who are at risk for developing ADHD generally carry some symptoms with them as early as preschool age and continuing throughout adolescence and even into adulthood. Attention-deficit/hyperactivity disorder is sometimes diagnosed in preschoolers, who display extremely high activity levels and impulsiveness. As a child grows into adolescence, his ADHD-associated behaviors may persist and become just as problematic as they were earlier in life. He may have difficulty concentrating, and be disorganized and easily distracted. Problems in adolescents with ADHD symptoms are likely to be expressed in different ways than they were in early childhood. Hyperactivity, for example, frequently takes center stage in early childhood but diminishes and may no longer be a problem by late adolescence or early adulthood. Inattention and impulsivity are likely to persist and can affect an adult's educational experience, work life, and relationships. Learning disabilities that were present during childhood also continue to exist in later years, as can any emotional, behavioral, and social problems that have not been fully resolved. (For more information about ADHD in adolescence, see Chapter 11.)

At one time or another all children and adolescents with ADHD may face some challenges relating to family relationships, status among their peers, social skills, academic achieve-

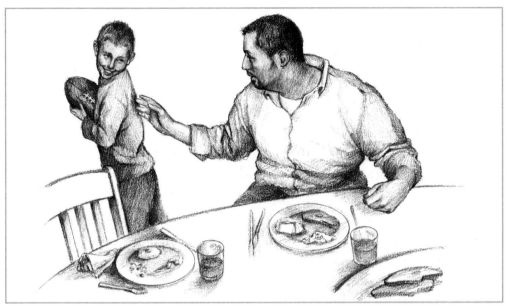

Often it may be difficult for your child to switch from one activity to another. Give your child advance notice before the start of new events (such as mealtimes) to help ease transitions.

ment, self-esteem, self-perception, and/or accidental injury. With help, however, children can learn to manage their symptoms in their early years as well as through adolescence and into adulthood. Early and accurate diagnosis is the first step toward organizing a plan that can make a difference to your child and your family.

As you begin to focus on the problems and issues that your child is facing, do not forget to appreciate and encourage his unique strengths and abilities as well, and to communicate that to him. A child with ADHD (like all other children) not only thrives on positive reinforcement and praise, but also desperately needs to know that his symptoms do not make him "bad," "undisciplined," "stupid," "unmotivated," or "lazy" as is so often implied. Educating him about what ADHD is—and what it is not—will help him cope with whatever discouraging comments or self-doubts come his way. The more he understands, the greater are his chances of success.

Finally, children with ADHD frequently grow up to become successful and happy adults. In the chapters that follow you will learn how to identify, treat, effectively parent, and advocate for your child in ways that will help him minimize his challenges and fulfill his enormous promise.

A PARENT'S STORY

Missed Clues and Lost Opportunities

"I suspected from my son's preschool days that he might have ADHD—not because of his activity level but because he could never stay focused on a single activity and he tended to forget things he had just learned. To me it was obvious that he was having real problems, but his teachers did not believe me because he is also unusually bright. They assumed that his restless behavior and underachievement were a result of 'just being bored.'"

"It was only in middle school, when my son began forgetting homework assignments, not taking notes, and even forgetting to take home books that he needed for homework from one day to the next, that his teachers began to think something serious might be going on. I remember one day when I was at the school for a parent-teacher conference, I saw him standing in the hall looking confused. I asked him what was wrong, and he told me he'd forgotten how to get to his next class. He did not know what to do or where to go."

"That was the day I decided to have him evaluated by a specialist. He was diagnosed with ADHD and is being treated now. His situation has improved, but I wish we had done this earlier before he fell so far behind. It is a huge relief to him, at least, to know that the problems he had been having at school were not his fault but were symptoms of his condition. My biggest hope for him is that he realizes the potential he had when he was born."

Roberta, Pittsburgh, PA

Chapter 2

Does My Child Have ADHD?
Evaluation and Diagnosis

If only it were as clear-cut to diagnose attention-deficit/hyperactivity disorder (ADHD) as it is to diagnose diabetes. Unfortunately, this is not the case because of some important differences. First, the line between having or not having diabetes is simple because the diagnosis can be confirmed through laboratory tests. In addition, the symptoms of diabetes are not easily confused with routine concerns in children who are well. As you will learn in this chapter, neither of these advantages exists in determining whether a child has ADHD.

No laboratory tests—no urine, blood, x-ray, or psychological analysis—can prove objectively whether ADHD is present. To complicate things further, the symptoms that characterize ADHD—inattention, hyperactivity, and impulsivity—occur in most children from time to time. Deciding whether a child's behaviors signal the presence of ADHD is therefore a complex process that involves comparing a child's behaviors and abilities to function with those of other children his age. To do this, pediatricians and mental health professionals must rely on parents' and caregivers' observations of how the child is functioning, information obtained from a child's teachers or other school professionals, and the results of well-designed questionnaires and interviews structured to evaluate whether specific problems may be interfering with a child's life on a daily basis. A diagnosis based on these types of evaluation procedures can become even more challenging when, as is often the case, other problems exist such as vision or hearing deficiencies, emotional disorders, or learning disabilities. An evaluation may require a team of professionals with different specialties because some of the accompanying problems are more medical in nature, some are more psychological, and others are related to learning and language processes.

Fortunately, many professional organizations, including the American Academy of Pediatrics (AAP), have developed guidelines in recent years that standardize the evaluation process for ADHD. As a result, diagnosis of the condition has become more consistent. In this chapter you will learn how a child is evaluated for ADHD, from the first recognition that "something may be wrong" through a methodical assessment of all of the specific problems that need addressing. Along the way you will find information about

- The types of behaviors that often alert adults to the possible presence of ADHD in children
- How your child's pediatrician will evaluate him and arrive at a diagnosis
- How your child's particular subtype of ADHD will be identified
- How clinicians will pinpoint the presence of any accompanying conditions
- How a "team approach" that involves you, your child, his educators, and his clinicians all working together can bring about the best diagnosis and prepare you for planning a course of treatment. One model for a team approach that can be an optimal approach as you and your family address the challenges posed by ADHD is called the medical home.

  A medical home includes
  – A partnership between your family and your child's primary care clinician
  – A relationship based on mutual trust and respect
  – Connections to supports and services to meet your child's and family's needs
  – Respect for your families cultural and religious beliefs
  – After-hours and weekend access to medical consultation about your child
  – Families who feel supported in caring for their child
  – Your primary care clinician working with your team of other care providers

Having a medical home available allows you to become a partner in being your child's "care manager," instead of having to take responsibility for this alone. (For more information about the medical home, see pages 97–98 in Chapter 5.)

Early Warning Signs: When ADHD Is First Suspected

Most experts agree that the tendency to develop ADHD is present from birth, yet ADHD behaviors are often not noticed until children enter elementary school. One reason for this delay is the fact that nearly all preschool-aged children frequently exhibit the core behaviors or symptoms of ADHD—inattention, impulsivity, and hyperactivity—as part of their normal development. As other children gradually begin to grow out of such behaviors, children with ADHD do not, and this difference becomes increasingly clear as the years pass. School settings can highlight a child's problems relating to inattention, impulsivity, and hyperactivity because classroom activities demand an increased amount of focus, patience, and self-control. These types of demands are not as prevalent at home or in playgroups, so in those settings, the child may have had fewer problems.

Usually by the time a child with ADHD reaches age 7 years, his parents have already become aware that their child's inattentiveness, level of activity, or impulsiveness is greater than is typical. You may have noticed that your child finds it nearly impossible to focus on a workbook for even a very short period, even when you are there to assist him. Or you may still feel as worn out at the end of a day with your overly active 8-year-old as you did when he was 2. Your child may ask adults questions so often that you have begun to suspect it is not "normal." Or, you may have noticed that he does not seem to be picking up the nuances of social interaction (respecting others' personal space, letting other people have a turn to talk) that his playmates are beginning to adopt. Yet it is difficult for a parent to tell whether such behaviors are just part of the normal process of growing up ("Plenty of six-year-olds get bored with workbooks!"), whether they are more frequently problematic because of parenting difficulties ("Maybe I've been too inconsistent with setting limits."), or whether this child's temperament puts him far to one end of the spectrum ("He's always been a handful."), but not so far as to represent a disorder such as ADHD. This is why, for a child to be diagnosed with the disorder, the AAP advises pediatricians to gather information about the child's behavior in at least one other major setting besides his home—including a review of any reports provided by teachers and school professionals. By comparing the child's behavior across 2 or more settings, the pediatrician can begin to differentiate among such varied reasons for attentional problems as a "difficult" but normal temperament, ineffective parenting practices, inappropriate academic setting, and other challenges. She can also clarify whether the child's behavior is preventing him from functioning adequately in more than one setting—another requirement for diagnosis.

"SOMETHING'S NOT RIGHT…"

What Parents Notice When ADHD Behaviors Emerge

It is sometimes hard to match the behavior we observe in our children with the formal terms used by pediatricians and other medical professionals. We rarely think of our children as having "hyperactive-impulsive problems." Instead, we think, "Why can't he ever settle down?"

To confuse matters, the terms that doctors use for these behaviors have changed in recent years. The term "ADD" (attention deficit disorder) was once commonly used, and referred primarily to the form of ADHD with "inattentive only" symptoms. These children are not overly active, and their symptoms may even go unnoticed by many adults because their behavior is not disruptive. But more recently, the umbrella term "ADHD" is typically used when describing all types of ADHD.

When reviewing the list that follows of typical remarks made about children with ADHD, ask yourself how many times per day or week you say or think the same things yourself. It is true that all parents make such comments now and then, but parents of children with ADHD continue to see the same behaviors on a daily basis, and for extended periods—long after other children have progressed.

Parents of Children With Predominantly Inattentive-Type ADHD Say

- "He seems like he's always daydreaming. He never answers when I talk to him. I wonder if he hears me."

- "He loses everything. I've had to buy four new lunchboxes since school started."

- "I'll ask him to go up to his room and get dressed, and ten minutes later I find him playing with his toys with only his shirt on."

- "He can't remember what he learns because he misses instructions and explanations in school. Even though we work so hard on his schoolwork at night, by the next day he's forgotten everything."

- "One teacher called him her 'space cadet,' and another her 'random student.'"

> ### "SOMETHING'S NOT RIGHT…" (CONTINUED)
>
> **Parents of Children With Predominantly Hyperactive/Impulsive-Type ADHD Say**
>
> - "He never slows down. You can never get him to sit down to finish a meal or get ready for bed."
>
> - "He interrupts constantly. You can't have a decent conversation when he's in the room."
>
> - "He never thinks before he acts. He knows he shouldn't run across the street before stopping to look, but he does it all the time."
>
> - "He operates out of order—like, 'ready…fire…aim.'"
>
> - "His classmates don't like him. He's always 'getting in their face.' No one invites him over to their house. He always has to be first and things always have to be his way."

First Steps Toward Evaluation

If you have begun to think that your child's poor progress at school, limited friendships, or frequent discipline problems add up to more than the typical difficulties of childhood, schedule an appointment with his teacher or school counselor as soon as possible. These people see your child daily in a group setting, where they can compare his behavior and ability to function to that of many other children his age. In many cases, teachers and counselors are trained to recognize symptoms of ADHD and similar disorders (although it is best not to assume that this is so). Certainly, they can give you a clearer idea of your child's experience at school, where ADHD so often manifests itself and creates problems. In many situations, it is the teacher or counselor who first notices that a child is failing to progress in ways that may indicate ADHD or a related disorder. In these instances, it is important for the teacher to contact the child's parents without delay to discuss the issue. Although teachers may identify more than 15% of their students as showing many of the behaviors compatible with ADHD and recommend those students for an evaluation by their pediatrician, a much smaller number of these students will actually be diagnosed with ADHD after a careful evaluation. Regardless of whether your child will end up being diagnosed with ADHD, it is important to follow up on teachers' concerns. The sooner a child with ADHD symptoms can be evaluated, diagnosed, and effectively treated, the greater his chances of progressing through school with good self-esteem and without losing too much ground.

If you and your child's teacher or other caregiver agree that your child is clearly having problems functioning in the areas of difficult-to-manage behaviors or learning at home or at school, make an appointment with his pediatrician to consider beginning an evaluation. Pediatricians are used to evaluating children for developmental or behavioral problems, and because ADHD is such a common problem, they often screen for it in school-aged children during routine health visits.

QUESTIONS YOUR CHILD'S PEDIATRICIAN MAY ASK YOU ABOUT SCHOOL

1. How is your child doing in school?

2. Are there any problems with learning that you or the teachers have seen?

3. Is your child happy in school?

4. Are you concerned with any behavioral problems in school, at home, or when your child is playing with friends?

5. Is your child having problems completing classroom work or homework?

Confirming the Diagnosis and Identifying Your Child's Specific Problem Areas

To create a uniform process for diagnosing ADHD among school-aged children, the AAP has created a list of standard guidelines for pediatricians to follow in evaluating a child reported to be inattentive, hyperactive, impulsive, underachieving academically, or having behavioral problems. These guidelines are based on a systematic review of the latest evidence about the prevalence of ADHD, coexisting conditions, and the diagnostic procedures most commonly used. You should expect your child's pediatrician to follow these recommended steps or a procedure much like them. The evaluation process will most likely require at least 2 or 3 visits to the doctor, possibly longer sessions with the pediatrician than you may be used to, and the filling out of a number of questionnaires, checklists, and other standard diagnostic tools. Your child's pediatrician may also ask you to forward questionnaires or ask the teacher to write a brief statement about your child's behavior and learning in the classroom before your first visit to make the initial interview more productive.

THE AAP RECOMMENDS...

Diagnostic Guidelines for ADHD

To ensure that children referred for evaluation for ADHD receive the most reliable, thorough assessment possible, the AAP has developed a set of diagnostic and evaluation guidelines, and recommends that pediatricians follow the steps outlined below. Your child's pediatrician may prefer one variation or another of a particular step (talking in person or on the phone with a teacher, or asking the teacher to write a brief narrative instead of or in addition to requesting written questionnaires), but in general each of these steps should be considered.

1. **Primary care clinicians should initiate an evaluation of ADHD for any child 4 to 18 years of age who has significant academic or behavioral problems and symptoms of inattention, hyperactivity, or impulsivity.** Attention-deficit/hyperactivity disorder often becomes apparent when a child enters a structured school setting, but symptoms can emerge prior to kindergarten or may not be recognized until adolescence.

2. **To make a diagnosis of ADHD, primary care clinicians should determine that the *Diagnostic and Statistical Manual of Mental Disorders, Fourth Edition, Text Revision (DSM-IV-TR)* criteria have been met (including documentation of impairment in more than one major setting) with information obtained primarily from reports of parents or guardians and teachers.** The *DSM-IV-TR* is a manual published by the American Psychiatric Association that describes all mental health conditions in children and adults. Information obtained from parents, guardians, and caregivers should be the basis for determining if the *DSM-IV-TR* criteria are met (see box on page 25). A revision of the *DSM,* which will be called *DSM-V,* is being prepared and is expected to be released in 2013.

3. **In the evaluation of a child for ADHD, primary care clinicians should include assessment for other conditions that might occur along with ADHD, including emotional or behavioral (eg, anxiety, depressive, oppositional defiant, and conduct disorders), developmental (eg, learning and language disorders), and physical (eg, tics, sleep apnea) conditions.**

Your child's pediatrician will start by listening to your observations and experience with your child's behavior and the difficulties that you have observed him having, along with your explanations of why you think (or do not think) that they may be related to ADHD. In addition to examining written reports from teachers, school counselors, or caregivers, she may ask you to relate what you have been told about your child's behavior in school and in his other daily settings outside the home. In many cases, parents' and teachers' opinions about a child differ significantly. This is all right and not unexpected. Your child's pediatrician will be prepared for this possibility and will listen carefully to reports from both "camps." She may ask to speak with other adults in your child's life (your spouse or partner, former teachers, coaches, or others in your community) to gain a broader impression of the types of problems your child may be experiencing.

Do not be surprised if your child's pediatrician seems to rely much more on these reports than on her own observation of your child. Children with ADHD do not necessarily exhibit symptoms of the disorder while in the doctor's office, so she will not expect to see them. (Keep in mind that ADHD, an attentional disorder, usually manifests itself in routine or monotonous situations, and visits to the doctor's office tend to be stimulating and outside of a child's usual routines.) Likewise, though she will perform a physical examination, she will not rely on this to indicate whether ADHD is present because there are no physical findings that by themselves verify ADHD, but will look for signs of medical conditions that can be associated with symptoms of ADHD. Your physician will carefully review your child's and your family's medical history for ADHD, related disorders, and other medical conditions that can have ADHD-like symptoms. Because ADHD has been shown to run in families, the discovery that you or other relatives have experienced ADHD-specific or similar symptoms may help point the way toward an accurate diagnosis.

You should familiarize yourself with the behaviors associated with the core symptoms of ADHD. These are summarized in the box on page 23.

CORE SYMPTOMS OF ADHD		
Inattention Dimension	**Hyperactivity-Impulsivity Dimension**	
	Hyperactivity	**Impulsivity**
• Careless mistakes • Difficulty sustaining attention • Seems not to listen • Fails to finish tasks • Difficulty organizing • Avoids tasks requiring sustained attention • Loses things • Easily distracted • Forgetful	• Fidgeting • Unable to stay seated • Moving excessively (restless) • Difficulty engaging in leisure activities quietly • "On the go" • Talking excessively	• Blurting answers before questions are completed • Difficulty awaiting his turn • Interrupting/intruding on others

Once your child's pediatrician has collected as much information about your child as you can provide and taken a family medical history, she will move on toward the first of what may be a series of structured questions, checklists, and evaluative procedures to identify his specific problems. She may ask your permission to have your child's teacher speak to her and complete some rating scales as well. This should be encouraged because the best treatment program will begin from as complete a view of your child as possible in many life settings. Other medical or mental health professionals to whom your child's pediatrician has referred you may also administer parts of the evaluation.

The AAP advises health professionals to begin with determining whether your child's behaviors match those considered necessary for making the diagnosis of ADHD. The behaviors comprising the "diagnostic criteria" for ADHD are set out in the manual *Diagnostic and Statistical Manual of Mental Disorders, Fourth Edition, Text Revision (DSM-IV-TR)*, developed by the American Psychiatric Association. This manual is presently considered the gold standard for professionals who diagnose behavioral and emotional disorders. The *DSM-IV-TR* lists 9 typical behaviors that apply to each of 2 subtypes of ADHD:

predominantly inattentive type and predominantly hyperactive-impulsive type. A child whose symptoms are significant and match at least 6 of the 9 behaviors described for each subtype is at risk for and may be diagnosed as having that disorder. A child with 6 or more matches in both categories is at risk for and may be eventually diagnosed as having a third subtype of ADHD: combined type.

Children and adolescents can only be diagnosed as having ADHD if

- Some of their symptoms were present before the age of 7 years.
- The symptoms have been observed to interfere with the child's functioning in 2 or more major settings, like at child care or at school.
- The behaviors significantly impair the child's ability to function in academic or social situations.
- The symptoms cannot be accounted for by another condition, either physical or mental, such as head trauma, physical or sexual abuse, depression, substance abuse, or a major psychological stress in the family or at school.
- The symptoms have been present for 6 months or more, and are more pronounced than for most children at the same developmental level.

Of course, all children exhibit many of these behaviors some of the time. Still, by considering to what extent such behaviors interfere with the child's ability to function at home, in school, and in social settings, your child's pediatrician or other health professionals can begin to arrive at a better idea of whether ADHD is the best explanation for the problems. As you have learned, it is necessary to differentiate behavior that is age-appropriate from behavior that strongly suggests a full diagnosis of ADHD. As you and your child's pediatrician consider these detailed descriptions of different types of behavior, you can develop a better idea about whether his behaviors are typical for his age, represent problems that need to be addressed, or signal the likelihood of ADHD. Pediatricians and other experts rely on knowledge about how ADHD-type behaviors are expressed at different ages, as described in the following boxes.

DIAGNOSTIC AND STATISTICAL MANUAL OF MENTAL DISORDERS, FOURTH EDITION, TEXT REVISION (DSM-IV-TR)

The following symptoms are included in the *DSM-IV-TR* diagnostic criteria for ADHD:

Inattention

- Often fails to give close attention to details, makes careless mistakes in schoolwork or other activities
- Often has difficulty sustaining attention in tasks or play activities
- Often does not seem to listen when spoken to directly
- Often does not follow through on instructions and fails to finish schoolwork or chores (not due to oppositional behavior or failure to understand directions)
- Often has difficulty organizing tasks and activities
- Often avoids, dislikes, or is reluctant to engage in tasks that require sustained mental effort (such as schoolwork or homework)
- Often loses things necessary for tasks or activities (eg, toys, school assignments, pencils, books, tools)
- Is often easily distracted by extraneous stimuli
- Is often forgetful in daily activities

Hyperactivity/Impulsivity

Hyperactivity

- Often fidgets with hands/feet or squirms in seat
- Often leaves seat in classroom or in other situations in which remaining seated is expected
- Often runs about or climbs excessively in situations in which it is inappropriate (in adolescents or adults, may be limited to subjective feelings of restlessness)
- Often has difficulty playing or engaging in leisure activities quietly
- Is often "on the go" or often acts as if "driven by a motor"
- Often talks excessively

Impulsivity

- Often blurts out answers before questions are completed
- Often has difficulty awaiting turn
- Often interrupts or intrudes on others

Reprinted with permission from: the *Diagnostic and Statistical Manual of Mental Disorders. 4th ed. Text rev.* Washington, DC: American Psychiatric Association; 2000.

COMMON SYMPTOMS OF INATTENTION

Early Childhood (preschool and early school years)

- **Behavior within normal range:** Difficulty attending, except briefly, to a storybook or quiet task such as coloring or drawing.

- **Behavior signaling an inattention problem:** Sometimes unable to complete games or activities without being distracted, is unable to complete a game with a child of comparable age, and only attends to any activity for a very short period before shifting attention to another object or activity. Symptoms are present to the degree that they cause some family difficulties.

- **Behavior signaling the possible presence of ADHD, predominantly inattentive type:** The child is unable to function and play appropriately and may seem immature, does not engage in any activity long enough, is easily distracted, is unable to complete activities, has a much shorter attention span than other children the same age, often misses important aspects of an object or situation (eg, rules of games or sequences), and does not persist in various self-care tasks (dressing or washing) to the same extent as other children of comparable age. The child shows problems in many settings over a long period and is affected functionally.

Middle Childhood (later primary grades through preteen years) and Adolescence

- **Behavior within normal range:** May not persist very long with a task the child does not want to do, such as reading an assigned book or homework, or a task that requires concentration, such as cleaning something. Adolescents may be easily distracted from tasks that they do not want to perform.

- **Behavior signaling an inattention problem:** At times the child misses some instructions and explanations in school, begins a number of activities without completing them, has some difficulties completing games with other children or grownups, becomes distracted, and tends to give up easily. The child may not complete or succeed at new activities, has some social deficiency, and does not pick up subtle social cues from others.

- **Behavior signaling the possible presence of ADHD, predominantly inattentive type:** The child has significant school and social problems, often shifts activities, does not complete tasks, is messy, and is careless about schoolwork. The child may start tasks prematurely and without appropriate review as if he were not listening, has difficulty organizing tasks, dislikes activities that require close concentration, is easily distracted, and is often forgetful.

COMMON SYMPTOMS OF HYPERACTIVITY/IMPULSIVITY

Early Childhood (preschool and early school years)
- **Behavior within normal range:** The child runs in circles, does not stop to rest, may bang into objects or people, and asks questions constantly.
- **Behavior signaling a hyperactivity/impulsivity problem:** The child frequently runs into people or knocks things down during play, gets injured frequently, and does not want to sit for stories or games.
- **Behavior signaling the possible presence of ADHD, hyperactive-impulsive type:** The child runs through the house, jumps and climbs excessively on furniture, will not sit still to eat or be read to, and is often into things.

Middle Childhood (later primary grades through preteen years)
- **Behavior within normal range:** The child plays active games for long periods. The child may occasionally do things impulsively, particularly when excited.
- **Behavior signaling a hyperactivity/impulsivity problem:** The child may butt into other children's games, interrupt frequently, and have problems completing chores.
- **Behavior signaling the possible presence of ADHD, hyperactive-impulsive type:** The child is often talking and interrupting, cannot sit still at mealtimes, is often fidgeting when watching television, makes noise that is disruptive, and grabs toys or other objects from others.

Adolescence
- **Behavior within normal range:** The adolescent engages in active social activities (eg, dancing) for long periods, and may engage in risky behaviors with peers.
- **Behavior signaling a hyperactivity/impulsivity problem:** The adolescent engages in "fooling around" that begins to annoy others, and he fidgets in class or while watching television.
- **Behavior signaling the possible presence of ADHD, hyperactive-impulsive type:** The adolescent is restless and fidgety while doing any and all quiet activities, interrupts and "bugs" other people, and gets into trouble frequently. Hyperactive symptoms decrease or are replaced with a sense of restlessness.

Adapted from: Wolraich ML, Felice ME, Drotar D, eds. *The Classification of Child and Adolescent Mental Diagnoses in Primary Care: Diagnostic and Statistical Manual for Primary Care (DSM-PC) Child and Adolescent Version.* Elk Grove Village, IL: American Academy of Pediatrics; 1996.

Knowing that your child's behaviors meet criteria for ADHD does not necessarily pinpoint the areas that cause her the most difficulties in her day-to-day functioning. Yes, using the criteria for making the diagnosis is important, but establishing the ADHD diagnosis is just the first step. A second major aim of an evaluation is to describe the problems caused by the ADHD behaviors specifically enough that they can be translated into a treatment plan. (See Chapter 3.) Your pediatrician will ask specific questions of you and your child to determine "functional impairment"—that is, the condition's impact on her day-to-day life. The functional impairments associated with ADHD include difficulties interacting positively with family members; keeping friendships; problems with social skills, academic achievement, and   following household rules; issues regarding self-esteem and self-perception; and problems with accidental injuries. Your pediatrician's recommendations for a treatment program for your child will depend to a large extent on these functional difficulties, and they will become the main "targets" for treatment.

As you and your child's pediatrician work through these detailed descriptions of different types of behavior, your child's problem areas should become increasingly clear. Some of these may fall out of the usual difficulties expected as a result of ADHD alone. Pediatricians, parents, teachers, and other members of a child's support team must thoroughly consider other environmental, situational, and emotional factors that may be influencing or causing these behaviors.

Special Circumstances: Preschool Children

We now know that the diagnostic criteria for ADHD can be applied to preschool children and that these criteria can appropriately identify children with the condition. However, there are added challenges in determining the presence of key symptoms of ADHD in preschoolers. Remember the requirement that ADHD needs to be diagnosed in settings other than just at home. Preschool-aged children are not likely to have separate observers if they do not attend a preschool or child care program, and even if they do attend, staff in those programs may be less qualified than certified teachers to provide accurate observations.

Where there are concerns about the availability or quality of nonparent observations of a child's behavior, your physician may recommend that you and your spouse or significant

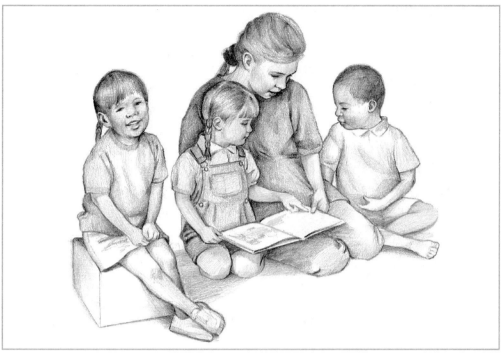

School settings can highlight a child's problems relating to inattention, impulsivity, and hyperactivity because classroom activities require an increased amount of focus, patience, and self-control.

other complete a parent training program prior to confirming an ADHD diagnosis for preschool-aged children. The parent training program should include you learning to identify age-appropriate developmental expectations and specific management skills for problem behaviors. Your pediatrician may then obtain reports from the parenting class instructor about improvement in behavior attained through the program. If you are in programs where your child is directly observed, instructors can report information about the core symptoms and function of the child directly. You might also consider placement in a qualified preschool program. Qualified programs include Head Start or other public prekindergarten programs. Preschool children displaying significant emotional or behavioral concerns may also qualify for Early Childhood Special Education (ECSE) services through their local school districts, and the evaluators for these programs and/or ECSE teachers may be excellent reporters around core symptoms of ADHD.

Is It Only ADHD, a Coexisting Problem, or Both?

One of the advantages offered by thorough discussions during the evaluation as well as diagnostic tests and rating scales that you, your child's teacher, and others complete is that they frequently pinpoint other emotional or developmental problems that exist alongside or in place of ADHD. As many as two-thirds of children with ADHD have one or more additional or coexisting conditions. The most frequent coexisting conditions include other behavior problems, depression, anxiety, learning disabilities, and language disorders.

Your child's pediatrician may be initially alerted to the possibility of some of these conditions by the reports you or other adults have provided. For example, a child described as frequently sad or irritable and who prefers isolated activities may be at risk for depression. A child who experiences frequent fears or unusual anxiety at being separated from a parent, and who has relatives with anxiety disorders, may have a similar disorder himself. Poor school performance may indicate a learning disability in addition to ADHD. Oppositional defiant disorder and conduct disorders are indicated by negative, disobedient, and oppositional behaviors toward authority figures and, less frequently, by a persistent violation of others' basic rights or of common social rules.

Coexisting conditions will be discussed in greater detail in Chapter 9. For now, though, it is important to consider the fact that such accompanying disorders

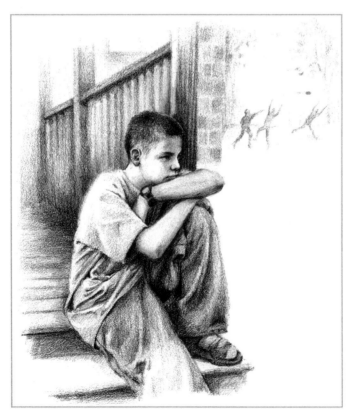

If your child seems frequently sad or prefers to be isolated, talk to your child's pediatrician for possible evaluation.

can have a profound effect on how well your child functions behaviorally, emotionally, socially, and academically. Your child's pediatrician and others working with your child should carefully consider whether such disorders may be your child's central challenge in his ability to function in his environment. To determine this, further evaluation, including referrals to other specialists, may be necessary. These evaluations can be part of the process to arrive at the most accurate diagnosis and treatment plan for your child.

The Importance of Teamwork

Evaluating a child for ADHD and related conditions is not an overnight, cut-and-dried process, nor can it be necessarily completed by your child's pediatrician or another professional alone. Arriving at a diagnosis of the problems or disorders causing them is an undertaking that requires the accurate observation, insight, experience, and even a certain amount of educated intuition on the part of parents, teachers, and medical professionals alike. As we described earlier (see page 16), the concept of the medical home is important in forming partnerships with care providers that can lead to more comprehensive and coordinated care for your child's ADHD. Also, a number of conditions that lead to behaviors similar to those resulting from ADHD must be considered and either eliminated or identified. The functional, real-world effects of each disorder must be carefully considered before an effective treatment plan can be put into place.

Assessing a child for ADHD requires patience and a great deal of teamwork from all adults involved—and this is good practice for the challenges to come. If the diagnostic process for ADHD seems complex, the process of choosing and implementing treatment may be even more so. For this reason, one of your foremost goals during this period should be to create and maintain clear lines of communication among the members of your child's diagnostic team. If you disagree with a teacher's assessment of your child's school performance, air your concerns now and work toward arriving at a better mutual understanding of some kind. Make sure that your child's pediatrician's findings and conclusions are reviewed with you in detail. This can avoid misunderstandings or unnecessary concerns about diagnoses, labels, or future recommendations. Pursue any questions that you still have. A low comfort level with any of the evaluation or diagnostic information you have received can be the biggest obstacle for you in deciding to begin, develop, and carry out a treatment plan for your child and your family. Keep teachers' reports, evaluation reports, and other materials used for diagnosis together in one file so that you can easily present and review them when necessary. The more professionals you see, the more important it is for you to have your own complete home-based medical record.

Diagnosis is only the first step in a long journey that you and your child are undertaking. By making sure that your child's support team is in agreement and that you are all focusing on the important issues, you can look forward with greater confidence to the day when his situation will be improved.

Q & A

Q: *I have ADHD, but because I have usually done well in school I was not diagnosed until I went to college, when my inability to keep to the task at hand began to seriously interfere with my school performance and relationships. As a child, I was quiet and shy, and because I did not have the hyperactive type of ADHD, no one noticed my condition. Now I am concerned that my daughter, who is in kindergarten, may have the same form of ADHD. But her teacher says she's doing well in school and has the usual number of friends even if she does have more trouble paying attention than most of her classmates. The teacher has discouraged me from having my daughter evaluated. Should I follow her advice?*

A: Children with inattentive-type ADHD are often first identified when the work demands of school start to accelerate—by third or fourth grade. Similar to your own experience, girls are often identified late, or not at all. You have a head start on this by already knowing a good deal about ADHD. The question now is whether your daughter's behaviors are still in the broad range of typical for a girl in kindergarten or whether they are an early expression of ADHD. The positive news from her teacher is that she is doing well in school and with social situations. An evaluation should be considered at any point that her behaviors start to interfere significantly with her school progress or other areas of functioning. As you suggest, ADHD does tend to run in families, so it is especially important to keep carefully tracking your daughter's progress. At this stage you might just want to bring your concerns to your child's pediatrician so that you can both keep a watchful eye on the situation and actively screen for problems at regular intervals.

Q: *My son has just been referred for assessment for ADHD. My neighbor tells me that her teenaged daughter was diagnosed with ADHD as a child and treated with stimulants for years, and then they found out that she had a learning disability instead. How can I tell if my child's problems are due to ADHD and not some other problem?*

A: Situations like this are the reason that the AAP and other professional organizations suggest that evaluations for ADHD follow a standard format and look at a broad range of areas of functioning instead of just ADHD itself. Estimates are highly variable, but a significant number of children who have been diagnosed with ADHD also have learning disabilities and, similarly, a significant number of children who have been diagnosed with learning disabilities also have ADHD. This is also true for other conditions, like oppositional defiant, conduct, anxiety, and depressive disorders, and emphasizes the importance of the AAP guideline recommendation that the evaluation of a child with ADHD should include assessment for coexisting conditions.

Q: *My son who is in fourth grade has just been diagnosed with ADHD. Both his teacher and doctor agree. I also agree that he is overactive and has trouble focusing. He is starting to have problems with his schoolwork and friendships even though he is a very bright and loving child. I can see that he needs some help, but I am also very concerned about his getting "labeled" and what negative effects this might have on him.*

A: You share a common concern of many parents whose child has just received the diagnosis of ADHD. In a sense, the diagnosis just tells you what you already know—that the problem behaviors you described during your child's evaluation match the diagnostic criteria for ADHD, and that they are causing your child significant problems on a daily basis. The diagnosis may serve as an entrance point for receiving different levels of help at school, and for knowledgeable teachers as a means to better understand and help your child. However, the diagnosis can be misunderstood by under-informed teachers or other adults who interact regularly with your child—but there is now a good deal of effort going into training teachers about ADHD and related disorders. You and your child's pediatrician can also contribute a great deal to this effort with your child's own teacher in many positive ways. Community support groups like CHADD (Children and Adults with Attention-Deficit/Hyperactivity Disorder) can provide you with a forum for discussing this and a place to meet parents who have already had experience with many of these challenges (see Resources on page 311).

Chapter 3

What Should We Do?
Treatment Options

"It was a shock, even after all the interviews, evaluations, and reports, when Andy was diagnosed with ADHD," writes a parent about her experience with her 8-year-old son. "On the one hand, I was so relieved to have an explanation for Andy's behavior. On the other, I was concerned that now the teachers and kids at school would 'label' him in negative ways. I was also worried about whether medications might be prescribed for him. I wondered, too, how Andy would respond to the diagnosis—would he lose even more self-confidence now that he knew he had a disorder?"

If your child has been diagnosed with attention-deficit/hyperactivity disorder (ADHD), you have probably asked similar questions and experienced some of the same concerns. You may also face a variety of responses to plans for your child's treatment—and much conflicting advice—from friends, relatives, educators, your partner, and even your child. Friends who have not been educated about ADHD may insist that your child's behavior is just the result of a discipline or parenting problem. You may feel that teachers who have witnessed the positive effect of stimulant medication in many children with ADHD are pushing you to put your child on the same type of medication. Your spouse or partner may believe that an alternative treatment is the answer, while your child insists that he does not have a problem at all—that others' concerns about him are "their problem."

Such opinions and concerns are understandable given how much inaccurate information about ADHD has been spread through the media, the Internet, and other channels, and it is important that it be addressed. In this chapter and the next one, you will find the responses to many of the questions that you and others are likely to have regarding treatment for your child. You will learn

- Which types and combinations of treatment programs have been shown to be most effective for ADHD

- How you, your child, his teachers, his pediatrician, and other members of his "treatment team" can work together to identify specific problem areas—"targets"—that will become the focus of treatment efforts
- How the treatment team can then create a management plan to address these target areas
- How ongoing observation and follow-up meetings of the treatment team can be used to monitor your child's progress and adjust aspects of his treatment when necessary to better address his ongoing needs
- How to help your child understand the treatment plan and become a member of the treatment team at each stage of his development

---

WHAT SHOULD I TELL THEM?

As you move from an ADHD diagnosis toward the creation of a treatment plan, you are likely to face a number of questions and remarks from friends, relatives, teachers, and others. Following are some responses that may help you and your child through awkward situations and answer some of your own questions.

"I have had several students with ADHD in my classes in the past. I recommend that your child be put on medication as soon as possible."

Response: "My child's pediatrician tells me that the most effective treatment plans, which may or may not include medication, need to be designed through a team approach by her, my child, us, and you, his teacher. Your feedback and observations are essential as we start the treatment process. If we make the decision to use medication as a part of the overall treatment plan, your observations and comments will be critical to monitoring and refining it."

"Everyone knows that ADHD is just a teacher's excuse to have kids "medicated" so they stay quiet and the classroom is easier to manage."

Response: "ADHD is a recognized disorder, it is widespread and it is treatable. Medication is just one of the ways that children can be helped to display fewer behavioral challenges and have more self-control from the teacher's perspective—but equally important is its ability to help children attend to daily tasks and thus function better."

WHAT SHOULD I TELL THEM? (CONTINUED)

"I don't care what the doctor says. There is no way you should give your child drugs."

Response: "First of all, the use of the word 'drugs' may not be the most appropriate choice when talking about medications for ADHD. It can be fraught with misunderstanding and negative implications, leading some parents to think their child is better off without taking anything. But in fact, stimulant medications for ADHD have been shown to make an enormous positive difference in the lives of many children. Some experts compare medication for ADHD as equivalent to prescribing inhalers for children with asthma—they regulate the child's system enough to allow him to carry on a normal life. Before making up our minds about treatment, we will talk to experts in the field, look at the research, read to inform ourselves, talk to other families whose children have been diagnosed with ADHD, and discuss our child's situation with him and with his doctors."

"He just seems depressed to me. How do you know it's ADHD and not some other problem?"

Response: "It's true that a number of other conditions (for example, anxiety disorder and depression disorder) can mimic some ADHD symptoms, but the evaluation my child just completed was designed to eliminate or identify most of them. Some children may have depression or anxiety disorders along with ADHD. Some of the rarer coexisting conditions, such as bipolar disorder, may start out looking identical to ADHD and only evolve into the specific disorder at an older age. That's why we'll continue to monitor and review his symptoms throughout childhood to make sure the diagnosis and treatment are still correct, timely, and appropriate."

"There's nothing wrong with me. It's other people who have a problem. My behavior is fine—they just can't handle it!"

Response: "I can see how hard it is on you when you feel like your teacher is always singling you out and picking on you, and when we always seem to be arguing about following rules at home. Now that we are finished with your evaluation, we can start learning more ways to turn these things around and make a happier situation at home and school."

Taking Action: First Steps in Developing a Treatment Plan

Treating ADHD is not like treating diabetes and other disorders, where drawing the line between children who have or do not have the diagnosis is clear, and where only children with the diagnosis have problems and need treatment while others do not. Attention-deficit/hyperactivity disorder is referred to as a "dimensional disorder," meaning that it occurs in varying intensities on a continuum, from children displaying some problem behaviors falling short of meeting criteria for diagnosis, to mild to moderate to severe. But there are no firm cutoff points on precisely what constitutes ADHD and what doesn't, and there are no definitive diagnostic tests for ADHD like there are for diabetes and many other disorders.

Many children, of course, have difficulty paying attention, controlling impulses, and being fidgety. Even when these problems do not initially seem to warrant the diagnosis of ADHD, your child's pediatrician may still suggest a number of measures as part of the evaluation and management: pediatric counseling, education about the range of normal developmental behaviors, home behavior management tools, school behavior management recommendations, social skills work, and/or help with managing homework flow and with organization and planning. If the symptoms begin to significantly interfere with your child's functioning at home and school on a daily basis, she will work with you to create a more comprehensive and organized overall plan. That plan may include the measures mentioned previously, but once the diagnosis of ADHD is made the plan may also include recommendations for medication management, behavior therapy, and other forms of treatment and support—all coordinated through an individualized and specific treatment plan.

While the core symptoms of ADHD (inattention, hyperactivity, and impulsiveness) are often the initial focus when a treatment plan is designed, the focus will then shift to the "functional disabilities" that parents and teachers were concerned about when they first sought help, such as schoolwork production, difficulty adhering to family rules at home, and challenges with maintaining friendships. These issues will become the "targets" for treatment. The American Academy of Pediatrics (AAP) has recently developed and updated a set of guidelines to assist pediatricians in developing comprehensive treatment plans for children with ADHD.

THE AAP RECOMMENDS…

Treatment Guidelines for ADHD

- Attention-deficit/hyperactivity disorder should be recognized as a chronic condition. A long-term treatment plan for children and adolescents with ADHD should be developed as for other children and youth with special health care needs (CYSHCN). Attention-deficit/hyperactivity disorder treatments can be effective for preschoolers through adolescents, but different considerations should be applied to children of different ages. Management of CYSHCN should follow the principles of the chronic care model and the medical home, which will be discussed below.

- Pediatricians should prescribe medications for ADHD approved by the US Food and Drug Administration (FDA) and/or scientifically sound parent- and/or teacher-administered behavior therapy as treatment for ADHD. Recommendations regarding the school environment, program, or placement may be part of the treatment.

- When medications are part of a treatment plan, clinicians should adjust doses of an FDA-approved medication for ADHD to achieve maximum benefit with minimum side-effects.

Adapted from: American Academy of Pediatrics. Clinical practice guidelines: diagnostic, evaluation and treatment of the child and adolescent with attention-deficit/hyperactivity disorder. In press.

ADHD as a Chronic Condition

Attention-deficit/hyperactivity disorder continues to cause symptoms and problems in day-to-day functioning in many individuals over long periods, and even when they are adults. It affects many areas of a child's life, and these areas need to be coordinated. The model for treating chronic conditions has been effective for other long-term problems, such as asthma and cystic fibrosis. Parents, children, and adolescents need a program for ongoing education about ADHD and related issues, and for adapting treatments to their needs over time. The treatments presently available address symptoms and functioning but are not curative.

The Medical Home Model

The medical home model has been accepted as the preferred standard of care for chronic conditions like ADHD. The medical home model recognizes that appropriate care for ADHD requires attention to multiple areas of a child's and family's life, including home, school, friendships, health care, emotional care, self-esteem, etc. This kind of care needs to be coordinated in all aspects to be the most effective, and parents and children need to be partners in an overall treatment plan with physicians, teachers, therapists, and other key individuals. In this model, all parties work together to identify specific goals or "target outcomes" on which to base decisions about treatment. In the medical home model the care that is provided to children and families is accessible, continuous, comprehensive, family-centered, coordinated, compassionate, and culturally effective, and addresses care needs at all levels. The care includes partnering with parents in

- Providing information about the condition to parents and children
- Updating and monitoring family knowledge and understanding on a periodic basis
- Counseling families about how they respond to ADHD
- Providing appropriate education to the child about the condition appropriate to their level of understanding, with updates as the child grows
- Having the pediatrician available to answer family questions
- Ensuring coordination of health and other services like education and behavioral treatments
- Helping families set specific goals in areas related to the child's condition and its affect on daily activities
- Linking families with other families with children who have similar chronic conditions as needed and available
- Working in collaboration with mental health clinicians if the child requires a consultation
- Addressing transition periods in the child's life and developing a transition plan as primary grade students transition to middle school, middle school adolescents transition to high school, and adolescents approach adulthood.

Identifying the Treatment Team

To successfully develop a treatment plan and put it into action, you will need to create a treatment team. This entails identifying the people most directly involved in your child's care and education. Their combined efforts will lead you to develop and carry out the most thoughtful, informed, and effective treatment plan. The team will obviously include you (the parent[s]), your child, your child's pediatrician, and your child's teacher. It may also include other adults at school and any involved mental health professionals. Why a team?

It will promote communication and the development of an agreed-on unified approach and, like all good teams, should be more valuable than the sum of each member's individual contribution to your child's success.

Creating a List: Defining Target Outcomes

Knowing that your child has been diagnosed with ADHD does not necessarily make the course of action for your child and family obvious. Before you, your child, his pediatrician, and other members of his treatment team can create an appropriate treatment plan, you will need to carefully consider which behaviors are most problematic for your child and most in need of attention. The best way to begin this process is to focus on his day-to-day problems with functioning at school, at home, and elsewhere—that is, to think in terms of *addressing your child's problems* in the context of your family and community resources, rather than *"treating his ADHD."* Such an approach involves first creating a full picture of your child—including all his strengths, problems, and accompanying diagnoses that were identified during his evaluation; a sense of how your family functions; a summary of any other major demands on family members that may affect his situation; the resources available in your community; and so on. Only in this broad context can your child's pediatrician decide with you how best to help create a realistic treatment plan that will work in your own unique circumstances. Once you have mapped out this broad picture of your child's situation and his difficulties functioning within it, your next step in creating a treatment plan is to initially identify 3 to 5 areas, goals, or targets that would most improve his functioning and self-esteem. Such targets may include

- Improved relationships with parents, siblings, teachers, and friends
- Fewer disruptive behaviors
- Improved academic performance, particularly in the volume of work, efficiency, completion, and accuracy
- Greater independence in self-care or homework
- Improved self-esteem and self-perception
- Safer behavior in the community (such as when crossing streets and riding bicycles, driving)
- More thinking before doing and making better behavioral choices

Once you, your child, and the other members of his treatment team have agreed on this list, you can turn these types of broad targets into specific behaviors and criteria that will help you know if your child is meeting the goals that you set. For example, if the broader area is "improved teacher relationships," your target outcomes might be

- Appropriately accepts feedback (no more than 2 arguments per day following feedback)
- Appropriately asks for adult help when needed (knows how to do the homework assignment before leaving class)
- Maintains appropriate eye contact when talking to an adult with fewer than 2 prompts to maintain eye contact
- Respects adults (talks back fewer than 2 times per period)
- Complies with 80% of teachers' requests with fewer than 2 noncompliances per period

Adapted with permission from: William E. Pelham Jr, PhD. School-Home Daily Report Card packet available for downloading at no cost at http://ccf.buffalo.edu. Also see American Academy of Pediatrics. *ADHD: Caring for Children with ADHD: A Resource Toolkit for Clinicians.* Elk Grove Village, IL: American Academy of Pediatrics; 2005.

Note how specific and countable each item has become. Also be aware that if you use words like "appropriately," you will need to define what it means for you, your child, your child's teacher, and other adults who will be involved with the treatment plan. After you have defined these targets, you can arrange them in order of priority to make sure that you are not taking on too much at once. Highest-priority issues will be those that most interfere with your child's functioning to the greatest degree at school, at home, or with his peers; those that impede his development; or those that have proved largely unmanageable so far. The extent to which a problem creates stress within your family may also affect the level of priority you give it. Your child's teacher can be an especially valuable contributor to this discussion because she observes your child daily within the context of an average range of same-aged children and thus may have a good idea of how disabling a particular behavior is.

Finally, it is important to review your target goals to make sure they are realistic within your child's and family's abilities to achieve and will result in improvement that can be observed and measured. Your child's pediatrician or other medical professional will be able to advise you on which goals are realistic and what types of results you can reasonably expect from which types of treatments. Expecting all "As" on your child's next report card may not be a realistic expectation no matter what treatment is chosen, but changes from "Ds" to "Bs" in certain academic subjects may be realistic and possible.

One of the greatest risks children with ADHD face is the loss of self-esteem as they experience academic failure, teasing from peers, and other upsetting effects of their inability to manage their behavior. Setting the bar a bit lower than ideal as you create a first set of goals will make it easier for your child to succeed, may give him a boost in confidence at a critical moment, and will ensure greater success down the road.

Involving Your Child

Once your child's target outcomes have been identified, placed in order of priority, and screened for feasibility, take a moment to make sure that he understands them as fully as possible given his level of understanding. *Treatment for ADHD should never be a process that is done to your child, but one that is as much as possible implemented by him with your support, guidance, and educated assistance as well as support from the rest of his treatment team.* For any treatment plan to succeed, your school-aged child or adolescent needs to understand the nature of ADHD, think and talk about ways in which he would like to improve his functioning, and feel comfortable participating in the treatment process to the extent that he is able. Your child should be present whenever possible for at least part of meetings that concern him, and parts of the discussion should be addressed directly to him at his level of understanding. Adolescents may also benefit from time alone with their doctor without parents present. Your child's reports on his day-to-day experiences with issues related to ADHD should be listened to and carefully considered. His prioritizing of ADHD-related problems should be taken seriously and addressed. By teaching him to consider his strengths, obstacles, and abilities to function in different situations and to monitor any changes, you are helping him prepare for the day when he will be in charge of his own care.

Becoming the Care Manager

Identifying target outcomes is only the first step, but an important one. Even though your child's pediatrician, teacher, and psychologist will take the primary responsibility for coordinating many aspects of his care from time to time, as your child's parent you should still expect to serve as the primary overall coordinator. In a medical home model, you would

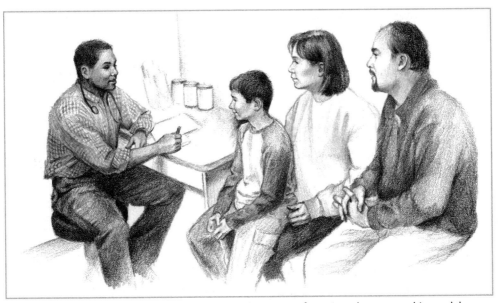

Your child should be present whenever possible for at least parts of meetings that concern him, and the discussion should be addressed to his level of understanding.

ideally partner with a care manager and all those who are caring for your child to success-fully coordinate the treatment plan. As time goes on you will need to take on many func-tions of care management—soliciting teachers' comments; providing your own observations and feedback; reviewing new evaluation results with medical personnel; staying informed on ADHD-related research; and seeking out the emotional and behavioral support that you, your child, and other family members need. The more thorough and active you are in coordinating this care among the team members, the more organized your child's treat-ment is likely to be. Many of the details of this role are discussed in Chapter 5 (see pages 97–98).

What Works and What Does Not—What We Know About Treatment

Once you, your child, and the treatment team have identified the target outcomes you hope to achieve, it is time to create a treatment plan to address those goals. With the help of the professionals on your treatment team, you will need to educate yourself on the various treat-ments that are available and what effects and limitations each is likely to have. (Reliable information on these topics is available in these pages and from other sources recommended in the Resources section on page 311.) As you begin to make decisions regarding treatment, keep in mind a central fact about treatment for ADHD: Nothing is written in stone. Because ADHD symptoms tend to change over time, your child may have different target outcomes at different stages of life and require different types of treatment. (What worked well during third grade may not work for fourth grade.) Because individual children respond to different therapies in a variety of ways, it may take several tries before you find a treatment program that works well. For all of these reasons, your child's treatment plan will consist of an ongoing process of treatment decisions, observation, review and, in most cases, treatment revision.

Choosing One or More Types of Treatment

In the years since ADHD symptoms were first described, a variety of treatment approaches have been tried and tested for their effectiveness. Only 2 of these approaches—use of medication and behavior therapies (a set of systematic, consistent techniques that parents and teachers can use to help a child better manage his behavior)—have been shown in well done studies to have consistent positive effects. The key is to find a balance between medication and behavior therapies—using the medication recommended by your pediatrician, as well as relying on behavioral management techniques that will help address behaviors such as tantrums and oppositional behavior (also see page 126). These approaches are often most effective when used in combination (see page 47).

Medical professionals and other experts have also studied traditional psychotherapy, special diets, nutritional supplements, biofeedback, allergy treatments, vision training, sensory integration therapy, chiropractic, and many other methods. Most of these approaches have either not been studied adequately enough to be recommended or have been shown to have minimal or no long-term effect. Some will be discussed in more detail in Chapter 10. The following table summarizes the most proven treatments for ADHD and accompanying problems.

THE EVIDENCE SHOWS	
Treatment For	**Possible Treatments[a]**
ADHD as a chronic condition	• Education for parents and treatment • A team approach among all of the child's caregivers, including parents and pediatricians (the kind provided in the medical home concept) • Empowerment of children and adolescents to "own" and help carry out their own treatment plan • Careful setting and monitoring of treatment targets, goals, and plans
Core symptoms of ADHD (inattention, impulsivity, hyperactivity)	• Stimulant medication (first-line treatment) • Proven behavior therapies • Atomoxetine, or bupropion (second-line treatment) • Individualized Education Program (IEP) based on Section 504 of the Rehabilitation Act or Individuals with Disabilities Education Act legislation

Oppositional and defiant behavior and serious conduct problems	• Behavior modification and management techniques
	  - Parent training
	  - School behavioral programs
	• Medication management if appropriate
	• IEP based on behavioral needs that cannot be met in the context of a regular classroom

Depression, anxiety, and problems with self-control and anger management	• Cognitive-behavioral therapy • Selective serotonin reuptake inhibitor or other antidepressant medication management if appropriate
Significant difficulties in family functioning	• Family therapy

Underachievement and learning and language disorders	• School IEPs that include
	  - Educational management
	  - Optimizing the classroom environment
	  - Addressing individual learning and language abilities and learning style

[a]These treatment options will be described in detail in chapters 4 through 7 and 9.

An Overview of Medication and Behavior Therapy for ADHD— The Mainstays of a Treatment Plan

Stimulants (such as methylphenidate and dextroamphetamine) have been the widest and best studied of any group of medications for the behavioral and emotional problems faced by children. Taken as recommended, they are effective and safe for most children with ADHD. Side effects mostly occur early in treatment, tend to be mild and short-lived, and in most situations can be successfully managed through adjustments in the dose or schedule of medication.

Parents are often confused by the fact that *stimulants* are the most frequently prescribed medications for ADHD. Why use stimulants, they wonder, when their child seems already overactive and overstimulated? The reason is that such medications are thought to work by "stimulating" the brain to keep slightly more of the brain chemicals (neurotransmitters) available that help all of us focus our attention, control our impulses, organize and plan, and stick to routines. With effective stimulant medication treatment, children with ADHD are better able to manage academic work and social interaction, attend to behavior modification techniques, and follow rules. Far from making a child someone he is not, as the word *drugs* implies, stimulants act as *medications* that can help many children with ADHD be who they are—with more appropriate attention, impulse control, and activity level.

The advantages and disadvantages of stimulant and non-stimulant medications will be discussed in greater detail in Chapter 4. For now it is important to consider that while many parents view placing their children on stimulant medication as a last resort—after all other measures have been tried—research has shown that such other treatments are more likely to work if the child is also taking stimulants. By helping the child focus, stimulants *lay the groundwork* for him to be able to respond better to behavior management techniques, academic instruction, and other demands on his attention.

Stimulant medication can be prescribed in a variety of doses and schedules. Because there has been so much controversy about ADHD in the media, many parents ask for and many physicians prescribe, the lowest dose of stimulant medication that leads to any improvement. It is now known that the best results from medication treatment are achieved by the dose that shows the *most* improvement with the least side effects.

Children with ADHD who have additional medical conditions or reasons why taking stimulant medication is not advisable may be prescribed non-stimulant medications instead, such as atomoxetine, guanfacine, tricyclic antidepressants, or bupropion. Children who were originally prescribed stimulants but experienced excessive side effects, improved for only very short periods, or responded insufficiently may also switch to non-stimulants. These non-stimulant medications have been shown to have variable degrees of positive effects on the core symptoms of ADHD. In general, non-stimulants have not been studied as extensively as stimulants, although more research into non-stimulants has been conducted in recent years. The strengths and weaknesses of this type of medication will be discussed more fully in Chapter 4.

Behavior therapy is considered another proven first-line treatment for ADHD. Behavior therapy emphasizes ways in which adults can better manage and shape their child's behavior by using sound behavior management principles and includes techniques for giving instructions and commands in a way that builds children's self-control and self-esteem. Programs that teach behavior therapy focus on how to give clear commands, use time-outs effectively, create effective rewards systems, and otherwise structure a child's environment in ways that work. Parents and teachers can learn to use these techniques effectively. This approach, which focuses on how adults can help children develop more appropriate and positive behaviors, has been shown to be effective, while child-focused approaches (such as traditional psychotherapy) have not. You will learn more about the specifics of behavior therapy in chapters 6 and 7.

Evidence for the effectiveness of behavior treatments in children with ADHD is derived from a variety of studies. The long-term positive effects of these treatments may be boosted when a chronic care model for child health has been implemented. Some of the more evidence-based behavioral treatments for children with ADHD (those with sound research behind them) follow.

EVIDENCE-BASED PSYCHOSOCIAL TREATMENTS FOR ADHD		
Treatment Type	**Description**	**Treatment Can Result In**
Behavioral parent training (BPT)	Behavior modification principles provided to parents for implementation in home settings	• Improved compliance with parental commands • Improved parental understanding of behavioral principles • High levels of parental satisfaction with treatment
Behavioral classroom management	Behavior modification principles provided to teachers for implementation in classroom settings	• Improved attention to instruction • Improved compliance with classroom rules • Decreased disruptive behavior • Improved work productivity
Behavioral peer interventions (BPI)	Interventions focused on peer interactions/relationships. These are often group-based interventions provided weekly and include clinic-based social skills training employed either alone or concurrently with behavioral parent training and/or medication.	When these treatments are provided in offices instead of schools, they have produced minimal effects. Interventions have been of questionable help in everyday life, even though they may be helpful in the groups themselves. Some studies of BPI combined with clinic-based BPT report positive effects on parent ratings of ADHD symptoms.

Adapted from: Pelham WE, Fabiano GA. Evidence-based psychosocial treatment for attention-deficit/hyperactivity disorder. *J Clin Child Adolesc Psychol.* 2008;37:184–214. Reprinted by permission of Taylor & Francis Group, http://www.informaworld.com.

Behavior therapy programs coordinating efforts at school as well as home may enhance the effects. School programs can provide classroom adaptations, such as preferred seating, reduced work assignments, and test modifications (location where tests are administered and time allotted for taking the test). Adolescents documented to have ADHD can also get permission to take college boards in an untimed manner by following appropriate documentation guidelines. These recommendations will be discussed further in Chapter 11.

The largest study of combined medication and behavioral long-term treatment for ADHD to date (known as the Multimodal Treatment Study of Children with Attention Deficit Hyperactivity Disorder [MTA], whose primary results were published in 1999) found that stimulants used as the sole form of treatment lead to significantly better results for the core symptoms of ADHD than behavior therapy used alone. A *combination* of the 2 approaches, however, has been shown to lead to the best overall improvement in several aspects of ADHD, especially when the areas of oppositional and aggressive behavior, social skills, parent-child relationships, and some areas of academic achievement are considered along with these core symptoms. The use of behavior therapy can also lower the rate of medication required in some cases. Parents in the MTA study whose children used this combined approach were often significantly more satisfied with the treatment plan than those whose children received medication alone. In this study, medication management and behavior treatment guidelines were carefully developed and followed. When the study guidelines were followed in this way, about 60% of children treated with medication alone could not be distinguished from their peers (who did not have ADHD) at the end of the 14-month study (which was a longer period than earlier, shorter studies). When children were treated with medication and the highly specific behavior treatments, this number increased to 70%. With this combination treatment, children with ADHD had fewer anxiety symptoms and fewer problems with academic performance and social skills.

After the initial 14-month study, the children returned to their own care from community providers but continued to be followed for 8 more years to track their progress. Changes in starting or stopping medication did not seem to be affected by whether they had been in the medication only, behavioral treatment only, or combined medication and behavioral treatment groups in the original study. Three patterns of outcomes were identified and remained consistent during the follow-up care: about one-third of children showed gradual improvement throughout the first 3 years and had more consistent use of medication at 3 years. About half of the children showed a large improvement at 14 months that was maintained at the 3-year follow-up. This group also had the best outcomes at 6 and 8 years, and this did not seem to be due to the extent of their medication use, but they were a less severe group initially. The third group, of about 15% of children, showed a large initial improvement followed by a trend of deterioration over time regardless of medication use. Children who continued to use medication over the 8 years of follow-up tended to have a minor decrease in their rate of growth for 2 years of medication treatment but then stabilized. However, no catch-up growth was found, although the follow-up reported to date does not take the children through their full growth period yet. It is not known what the outcomes would be if a group of children received the same careful treatment and medication adjustment that they had received in the 14-month initial study period. It is also unclear what the outcome would have been if these children had also received care according to the sound medical home principles discussed previously.

It is important to point out that all medication and behavior approaches are not the same—one size does not fit all. The most successful approaches, like those in the MTA study, are evidence-based—they have been carefully researched and found to work. Evidence-based approaches for the treatment of ADHD will be reviewed in the chapters that follow. More untested treatment approaches are not as reliable. For example, in the MTA study, only about 25% of the children treated with less rigorous approaches than the study used, even if they include the use of medication and some form of behavior management, did as well as their peers.

Other Components of the Treatment Plan

Other treatments, including psychotherapy and family or marital therapy, may provide valuable assistance to families who have problems that are not directly caused by but are related to and affect ADHD. The stress that a child's behavior may place on the family can prevent them from carrying out a treatment plan unless such issues are addressed. When one parent or partner also has ADHD (a frequent occurrence because the condition runs in families), this can put even more stress on family functioning.

The fact that ADHD symptoms frequently manifest themselves in school settings, and children with ADHD may also have learning disabilities and other learning-related conditions, means that academic intervention can make a difference for your child even if it does not directly affect her ADHD symptoms. Children with clearly diagnosed learning disabilities qualify for special education services in school. In this situation, schools are federally mandated to develop Individualized Education Programs (IEPs) that detail exactly what services will be offered and how they will be delivered. The same is true for children who have behavioral needs too severe to be handled in a regular classroom.

Fortunately, students who have learning or behavioral needs related to their ADHD symptoms but do not have diagnosed learning disabilities or such severe behavioral needs can also receive services (see Chapter 7). While such programs, strategies, and considerations do not directly address the core symptoms of ADHD, they support the child with ADHD academically and behaviorally and, thus, help maintain their success and self-esteem.

Clearly, because each of the treatments discussed targets different results, it is most common to use several types of treatment at any given time. While most children's treatment plans may begin with medication and behavior therapy, additional approaches, such as academic intervention, psychotherapy, and family therapy, may provide added support when they are indicated. When choosing from the menu of treatment options, you will need to consider whether

- You have the work schedule, time, confidence in the treatments, and energy necessary to adhere to them.
- They address one of your child's most important 3 to 6 target outcomes.
- The therapies are available in your community, which isn't always the case.
- Your family can realistically afford them, particularly since behavior therapy often isn't covered by health insurance.

Consider how good a match each of these approaches is for your child, and whether the results can be satisfactorily monitored. How smoothly can each treatment be combined with the others that you plan to implement? How available are these techniques or programs in your community? How long are the benefits likely to last after the treatment has ended? Are there any possible negatives or side effects? How well do the positive effects translate to your child's everyday life (are you still using the parenting techniques 3 days after the training session and are they helping with his behavior)? How well does the treatment method coincide with the values and goals of your family as a whole? Most importantly, how does your child feel about this type of treatment? Will he feel stigmatized by his friends or family because of it?

In the end, no matter how effective the other members of a treatment team believe a certain approach to be, it will most likely break down unless the child himself understands its purpose and is committed to making it work. For this reason, the litmus test for any mode of treatment should be whether it promotes your child's self-confidence, improved self-management, and higher self-esteem. It may take more than one try to create this type of treatment plan, and you should expect to be constantly reshaping it, but the potential benefits are worth the effort.

Follow-up Plan

Your pediatrician or other clinicians should periodically provide a systematic follow-up for children and adolescents with ADHD. One good model would be for a child to be initially seen by the pediatrician monthly once treatment is prescribed, and then every 3 to 4 months in the first year of treatment. The pediatrician should consult with parents, teachers, and the child about how well target outcomes are being met and what, if any, unexpected or negative effects have been experienced. Your input will allow the treatment team to further tailor the treatment plan in ways that can make it more effective. If the target outcomes are not met, the treatment team should reevaluate the original diagnosis, treatments used, whether the treatment plan is being carefully followed, and presence of any coexisting conditions (see Chapter 9).

SETTING A PLAN FOR YOUR CHILD'S FOLLOW-UP VISITS

The AAP recommends that physicians periodically provide systematic follow-up for your child. You can help structure each visit so that you and your physician can include as many of the following steps as possible.

1. Discuss and review your own observations of your child, his most recent teachers' reports, and the results of any rating scales completed since the last visit.
2. Share information about the target behaviors and how they might have changed since the last visit.
3. Review the plan agenda, the target behaviors, and the current methods of treatment.
4. Screen for new coexisting conditions.
5. If your child is taking medication, review any possible side effects.
6. Review your child's functioning at home, including his behavior and his family relationships.
7. Review your child's functioning at school, especially relating to academics, behavior, and social interaction. Make sure that some information is obtained directly from your child's teacher (particularly important before changing any medication dose).
8. Discuss your child's self-esteem, and review his behavioral, social, and academic self-management issues.
9. Assess and supplement your child's understanding of ADHD, coexisting conditions, and treatment as appropriate for his age.
10. Discuss any current problems relating to organizational skills, study skills, homework management, self-management skills, anger management, etc.
11. Make sure that you get all the information you need to enable you and your child to make informed decisions that promote his long-term health and well-being.
12. Review and revise your child's treatment plan.
13. Make sure that there is a system in place for communication among you, your child, his teacher, and the clinician between visits.

A PARENT'S STORY

A Team Effort

"At first I was surprised to hear from other families how often kids switched their medication or tried new doses or schedules," writes the father of a 9-year-old. "I guess my first reaction was, 'Don't the doctors know what they're doing? Why can't they get it right the first time?' After we started the treatment process, though, I found it very reassuring that Tina's pediatrician wanted our feedback on how the medication was working, and how we were doing with the behavior therapy. Tina experienced some irritability in between doses with her first prescription so we switched to a long-acting medication where she only had to take one dose per day. That worked a lot better, and then we figured out that working more in concert with her teacher on the behavior techniques improved the situation even more. As Tina started doing much better, she became more eager to participate in the plan. By the end of the first year I felt like we'd all worked as a team to put together the best program we could for her. It was great knowing we had all these people's support and that as Tina's life changed her treatment could change along with her."

John, Tampa, FL

Follow-up visits should cover all of the ground since your last visit. This includes sharing your own observations of your child's recent behaviors, ongoing problems, and new concerns and screening for any new coexisting conditions. You and your child should be given the opportunity to ask questions and should be informed about any major new research or other information pertaining to his condition or his treatment. The most recent rating scales, teachers' observations, and other progress reports should be reviewed. Finally, your child's target outcomes can be reviewed and, if your child is clearly not meeting the current goal for each one, his treatment can be reassessed.

If your child is not meeting his specific target outcomes, you, your child's pediatrician, and your child should consider the following issues:

- Were the target outcomes realistic?
- Is more information needed about your child's behavior?
- Is the diagnosis correct?
- Is another condition hindering treatment?

- Is the treatment plan being followed?
- Has the treatment failed?
- What coping strategies can you learn to deal with target behaviors that cannot be fully resolved through appropriate treatment?

No treatment for ADHD is likely to completely eliminate all of the symptoms of inattention, hyperactivity, and impulsivity and associated problems and conditions. Children who are being treated successfully may still have trouble with their friends or schoolwork. Still, you should see signs of progress relating to your child's specific target outcomes or general behavior. If not, your child's diagnosis and/or treatment should be revised. A revised diagnosis is not a sign of failure in you, your child, or his pediatrician. It is merely a signal that your child's treatment team has yet to create the optimal response to his symptoms.

Treatment of ADHD is in many cases largely a matter of continually monitoring and re-shaping the plan, and you can expect treatment to change as your child adjusts to treatment, grows, and develops over time. As these changes are made, continue to make sure that any and all treatments are aimed at fostering good self-esteem and that your child understands them to the extent possible given his developmental level. Follow-up visits should be geared in large part toward educating your child and empowering him to participate more and more in decision-making as he approaches adolescence. Adolescents who "own" their problems and treatment plans are much more likely to make progress. Those who feel that treatment changes are being "shoved down their throats" will naturally resist or abandon treatment and are at high risk for school failure, poor peer relationships, low self-esteem, substance abuse, and conduct problems.

Treatment for ADHD is generally considered to have failed only in cases when a child shows no response to appropriate trials and alterations in medication at maximum doses without side effects, when he cannot learn to control his behavior in spite of appropriate behavior therapy, or when a coexisting condition persistently interferes with the meeting of target outcomes. In each of these cases, the diagnosis would need to be carefully reconsidered and additional consultations might be appropriately called for. In treating, monitoring, and following up on treatment for your child with ADHD, communication is key. As treatment continues in one form or another throughout your child's early years, you will need to make sure that

- He understands and supports the goals and methods of his treatment.
- Other family members are equally informed and supportive.
- Teachers continue to work with him in effective ways and pass their observations on to him and you.
- Pediatricians and other medical personnel receive this feedback from you, his teachers, and others who spend time with your child.
- You and other members of the treatment team remain up to date on the legislation and medical, educational, and psychological issues that affect your child.

A child who knows as much as possible about ADHD will be better prepared as he faces challenges at home and school. A sibling who understands the steps involved in the treatment process may be more patient when you need to take time out for a parent training course. A pediatrician who is informed of any new family problems or stressors can make better decisions regarding treatment. Finally, educators who know that you and your child understand the nature of ADHD are often more eager to work together to manage it.

Attention-deficit/hyperactivity disorder is not yet curable, but it is certainly treatable. With attention, dedication, and a long-term outlook, you and your family may be able to look forward to continuing progress in the target areas you have defined.

Q & A

Q: *My son was recently diagnosed with ADHD, and we have worked out a treatment plan with his pediatrician. The problem is, the plan involves having my son take medication twice each day, implementing a number of new parenting practices, changing his homework habits, and dealing with the fallout with my other children and my wife. Frankly, since the diagnosis I feel like my entire family is falling apart. We can't seem to handle this responsibility on top of all of the pressures of daily life. Is there anything we can do to get better organized?*

A: The initial steps in starting and carrying out a treatment plan for ADHD can be stressful for all families. It is not at all unusual for a family undertaking a complex treatment program—learning to administer medication on time, consistently applying new behavior-modification techniques, and making and keeping appointments with various specialists—to feel at first that it is almost impossible to get through a single day. That is why it is so important to define a limited number of target goals and treatments that are achievable and can fit into your family's daily life. If the treatment plan overwhelms you and your child, the chances of it succeeding will significantly decrease. If the plans you make around these goals are successful, it will give you more energy to take on the next steps. Through all this, make sure that you keep your support systems in place—other family members, members of the treatment team, and community support groups. Also make sure that you emphasize more than ever the things that you and your family value and enjoy.

Q: *My 14-year-old daughter has recently begun treatment for inattentive-type ADHD. From the beginning, we have involved her in her own diagnosis and treatment and have asked for her input as we created a list of behavioral goals and put together a treatment plan. She is now responding well to treatment, but I'm not sure that she really comprehends the nature of her condition. She keeps asking us "When can I stop my medication?" and "Why does everyone say there's something wrong with me?" We know how important it is for her to understand and participate in her own care. What can we do to make this happen?*

A: Receiving a diagnosis of ADHD can be a blow for most children and adolescents, and some take longer than others to adjust in a positive way. That is why it is so important to involve children and adolescents in as many of the steps in evaluation and treatment as possible. Adolescents, particularly, do not want to stand out from their peers in any way, so obtaining buy-in to the target goals and treatment plan is especially important at this age. Part of the treatment for your daughter should include ways of keeping the diagnosis and treatment plan as private as she wants. This might include decisions (that she is part of) to figure out a medication schedule that does not involve taking medication at school, arranging for tutoring outside of school hours, etc. And, of course, the more good information she has about ADHD and its treatment at every stage the better.

Chapter 4

The Role of Medications

If your child has been diagnosed with attention-deficit/hyperactivity disorder (ADHD), you may be asked to consider using medication as part of his treatment plan. As we pointed out in Chapter 3, stimulant medications have been shown to provide a proven safe and effective way to manage the core symptoms of ADHD (hyperactivity, inattention, and impulsivity). Thus they are a first-line treatment recommendation for most children who have this condition—often in combination with behavior therapy and other forms of treatment. The use of stimulants has been compared to wearing glasses for a person with poor vision, because stimulants help "put things into focus" for a child when they are active in his system. As soon as the effects of the dose of stimulant wear off—or the glasses are taken off—things go just as out of focus again. Stimulants help children improve their functioning in measurable ways—just as glasses enable the child with poor vision to learn to read. But keep in mind that just as glasses can help focus but do not make a child a reader, so stimulants do not "make" a child perform better—he has to do that work himself.

It is one thing to understand how stimulants might help a child, but quite another to consider using this medication with your own child. You have probably heard of medications like Ritalin and Adderall, commonly known brand names for methylphenidate and amphetamine, respectively—just 2 members of the class of medications known as stimulants. The increase in the prescribing and use of stimulants over the last couple of decades has led to concerns in the media and among parents about whether stimulants are being overprescribed for children with ADHD. Yet even with that, the amount of medication presently taken by children does not seem to exceed the amount needed to treat carefully diagnosed cases of ADHD in the United States.

Most of this increase in stimulant medication use likely stems from better recognition and diagnosis of ADHD (including a greater awareness of ADHD in girls) and from the trend for children to be treated for longer periods, sometimes through adulthood. Nevertheless, some pediatricians still debate whether ADHD is overdiagnosed or underdiagnosed, and that is why you need to be careful about having an accurate diagnosis for your child before you even think about embarking on a course of medication management (see Chapter 2).

You learned in Chapter 3 that stimulants are presently considered effective and safe medications, and there are few situations in which they are medically inadvisable. However, they are not for everyone. A small number of children and their families will find that the side effects are too intrusive at the doses that are most effective for that individual child. Some parents may find that their own negative feelings about the medication, or some other issue within the family, prevent them from properly implementing this part of the treatment plan considering stimulant medication use. Non-stimulant medications are also available for the treatment of ADHD and will be discussed later in this chapter.

Ultimately, you and your family must weigh the pros and cons of choosing medication as part of the treatment plan for ADHD. The more educated you are about the medication process, the better prepared you will be to make this decision. In this chapter, you will learn

- What types of medication are approved to treat ADHD
- How your child's medication dose and schedule will be determined, monitored, and adjusted
- What types of medication other than stimulants are available to children with ADHD
- How to talk with your child about the use of stimulants or other medications
- How to make the most of the benefits that medications provide

---

A PARENT'S STORY

Missed Clues and Lost Opportunities

"Like most parents, I didn't like the idea of my 10-year-old child using stimulant medication to manage his ADHD. But I was very concerned about his behavior and ability to learn, and I felt we needed to do whatever was necessary to help him in those areas. We tried stimulants, and within the first few days we began to see an amazing difference. His concentration improved. He stayed focused on his tasks. We still had to try several different types of stimulants during that early period and adjust the dose a few times, but eventually he was able to retain what he had learned much better than before. Where there was once frustration, I began instead to see a happier and more confident child."

"Once I saw that medications could help him succeed, I felt we had made the right decision. When people ask me about stimulants now, I tell them they're a helpful treatment that gets a bad rap for reasons that now I don't entirely understand. Still, I think families rely too much on them sometimes. Parents still need to learn how to help their child improve his behavior, learn organizational skills, and take advantage of school support to figure out the best approaches to learning. Medication can help, but as I see now, that's mostly because the child and his family have also put in a lot of hard work."

Margaret, Sacramento, CA

What You Need to Know About Stimulant Medications

In Chapter 3 we explained that stimulant medications are thought to work by stimulating the brain to make available slightly more of the brain chemicals (neurotransmitters) that help our brain cells communicate more efficiently. This increased efficiency allows us to better focus our attention, control impulses, organize, plan, and stick to routines—leading to a reduction in the core ADHD symptoms of hyperactivity, inattention, and impulsivity. Parents of a child with ADHD who is taking stimulants may notice a decrease in the number of accidental injuries their child experiences as her impulsivity declines. They may also observe that her social relationships may improve as her intensity decreases, her social judgment improves, she responds more positively to others, and she is able to communicate more effectively. The significant improvement in the child's school behavior—sometimes to the point that it is indistinguishable from that of her classmates—is particularly satisfying to most children and their families. Children treated with stimulants for ADHD can also enjoy a longer attention span, an increased ability to stay focused on a task, and more productivity and accuracy in schoolwork.

Once again, stimulants are generally considered highly effective and safe medications. They are, though, categorized by the US Drug Enforcement Administration as Schedule II drugs—medications that have been approved for medical use but have a high potential for abuse in adults if they are not used properly. Because of this, the rules for prescribing stimulants may differ from those for other medications (such as antibiotics) from state to state. Although there is a lot of discussion in the media about the potential for the abuse of stimulant medications, they don't produce speed-like or euphoric effects in children or adolescents when used properly and restricted to normal treatment doses. In addition, the use of stimulants by children with ADHD has not been found to put adolescence at an increased risk for street drug use.

Stimulants work similarly in people who do and do not have ADHD—they can help most children and adults achieve better focus and concentration. Because of this, having a positive response to stimulants is not a test of whether a child has ADHD. Nor does needing a higher dose than another child mean that your child's symptoms are more severe. Doses vary with the individual regardless of the severity of symptoms. Some children with mild symptoms may need higher doses of medication while others with more severe symptoms require lower doses.

Medications can be described by their generic (chemical) names but are most often known to parents by their brand names. The 2 generic classes of stimulants proven to be effective for the treatment of ADHD are methylphenidate and amphetamines. The brand names of the methylphenidate preparations currently available to children with ADHD are Ritalin, Metadate, Methylin, Focalin, Concerta, and Daytrana. A number of different amphetamine medications are also available and include Dexedrine, Dextrostat, Vyvanse, Dexedrine Spansules, and Adderall.

Both classes of stimulants have similar effects and side effects. Different preparations also have different durations of action, as described in the table below. Comparing doses of different medications can be confusing to parents. The amount of each medication prescribed (in milligrams per dosage or per day) is unique to that particular medication—so, for example, 5 mg of methylphenidate (Ritalin) is only about half as strong as a dose of 5 mg of dextroamphetamine (Dexedrine).

FDA-APPROVED MEDICATIONS—DOSING AND PHARMACOKINETICS
First-line Medications Used in the Treatment of ADHD

Medications	Brands	Frequency of Use	Effect Begins (in minutes)	Effect Lasts (in hours)	Maximum Dose	Available Doses
Mixed amphetamine salts	Adderall	Once to twice a day	20–60	6	40 mg	5-, 7.5-, 10-, 12.5-, 15-, 20-, and 30-mg tablets
	Adderall XR	Daily in the morning	20–60	10	40 mg	5-, 10-, 15-, 20-, 25-, and 30-mg capsules
Dextroamphetamine	Dexedrine/ Dextrostat	Twice to 3 times daily	20–60	4–6	40 mg	5- and (Dextrostat only) 10-mg tablets
	Dexedrine Spansule	Once to twice daily	60+	6+	40 mg	5-, 10-, and 15-mg capsules
Lisdexamfetamine	Vyvanse	Daily in the morning	60	10–12	70 mg	20-, 30-, 40-, 50-, 60-, and 70-mg capsules

FDA-APPROVED MEDICATIONS—DOSING AND PHARMACOKINETICS (CONTINUED)

First-line Medications Used in the Treatment of ADHD

Medications	Brands	Frequency of Use	Effect Begins (in minutes)	Effect Lasts (in hours)	Maximum Dose	Available Doses
Methylphenidate	Concerta	Daily in the morning	20–60	12	72mg	18-, 36-, and 54-mg capsules
	Methylin	Twice to 3 times daily	20–60	3–5	60 mg	5-, 10-, and 20-mg tablets and liquid and chewable forms
	Daytrana	Apply for 9 hrs	60	11–12	30 mg	10-, 15-, 20-, and 30-mg patches
	Ritalin	Twice to 3 times daily	20–60	3–5	60 mg	5-, 10-, and 20-mg tablets
	Ritalin LA	Once daily	20–60	6–8	60 mg	20-, 30-, and 40-mg capsules
	Ritalin SR	Once to twice	60–180	2–6	60 mg	20-mg capsules
	Metadate CD	Daily in the morning	20–60	6–8	60 mg	10-, 20-, 30-, 40-, 50-, and 60-mg capsules
Dexmethylphenidate	Focalin	Twice a day	20–60	3–5	60 mg	2.5-, 5-, and 10-mg tablets
	Focalin XR	Daily in the morning	20–60	8–12	20 mg	5-, 10-, 15-, and 20-mg capsules

Abbreviation: FDA, US Food and Drug Administration.

As you can see from the table on page 64, these medications have variable durations of action: short-acting (around 4 hours), intermediate-acting (6–8 hours), and long-acting (10–12 hours). Short-acting preparations are very well studied and begin acting rapidly. The negative side is that they have to be taken 2 to 3 times each day to cover a 12-hour period. This can lead to forgetting doses, and many children do not like to be seen taking medication in school. Intermediate-acting preparations can span a school day, but won't be active for after-school homework. Some children on long-acting preparations have difficulty with decreased appetite in the evening and initial insomnia, which can also be a concern.

Short-Acting Stimulants

Different preparations may have different advantages. Methylin is a short-acting medication available as chewable tablets and oral solutions for children who have difficulty swallowing pills and capsules. Short-acting preparations are also used in children weighing less than 35 pounds, because sufficiently low doses exist for children of this weight. Short-acting doses may also be used to extend the hours of medication coverage. For example, if an intermediate-acting medication is given that lasts for 8 hours, a short-acting medication can be used when homework needs to be done in the evening. Also, short-acting medications can be given when a child wakes up to help reduce ADHD symptoms during the morning routine and then allow longer-acting preparations to be given right before a child leaves for school.

Longer-Acting Stimulants

Longer-acting stimulants are just as effective as the short-acting preparations, but limit the need for multiple doses during the day, and also decrease the stigma of having to take medication doses in school. Cost can be an issue as these medications are often more expensive than the short-acting forms. Sustained-release preparations with the stimulant suspended in wax (Ritalin SR, Metadate ER, Methylin ER) need to be swallowed whole to remain long-acting. Preparations using beads or pearls generally contain half of the beads to be released immediately and the other half as coated delayed-release bead medication. The products using this technology include Dexedrine Spansules, Ritalin LA, Focalin XR, Adderall XR, and Metadate CD. These beaded preparations are helpful for children who have trouble swallowing pills because the capsules can be opened and sprinkled into tea-spoons of apple sauce, yogurt, or other foods. These beads should not be chewed. Concerta is a long-acting preparation in a capsule with a pump technology that delivers one dose immediately and long duration components for the equivalent of 3-times-daily dosing. These capsules cannot be chewed. They also do not dissolve, so they can be found in chil-dren's stools. Daytrana comes as a patch. The medication is slowly absorbed through the skin, and the absorption may not reach a peak until 7 to 9 hours, and symptoms of ADHD may not become noticeably reduced until the end of the first 2 hours. Patches are helpful for children who can't tolerate any of the oral forms of stimulants. Timing during the day can be controlled by knowing that the medication action ends about 2 to 3 hours after the patch is removed. Some children develop skin rashes. There is some concern, as you will read in Chapter 11, about stimulants being sold and used for recreational purposes, or being abused by youth who have ADHD. Lisdexamfetamine (Vyvanse) is a prodrug. This means that it requires oral ingestion to be converted to the active drug, which may decrease the risk of abuse potential.

Studies have shown that each of these stimulants (methylphenidate or amphetamines) is potentially equally effective in treating the symptoms of ADHD. However, individual chil-dren may respond better to one particular stimulant or be limited, due to side effects, from taking another. This is why it is necessary to begin with one stimulant; monitor the dosing and results; and with your pediatrician's guidance, perhaps alter (or titrate) the dose or switch stimulants until optimal results are achieved. No laboratory tests, electrocardio-gram (EKG) monitoring, or psychological tests are routinely necessary for monitoring the use of these medications.

Another medication—called Strattera (atomoxetine)—is not a stimulant, but it is a medica-tion for ADHD that is approved by the US Food and Drug Administration (FDA). For more information about Strattera, see pages 77–78.

How Will My Child's Medication Treatment Be Determined?

The ease with which preparations can be administered and the minimization of side effects are important for the quality of life concerns that children, youth, and parents express around the decision to use medication. Other issues that should be taken into account include the time of day when the targeted symptoms occur, when homework is usually done, whether medication remains active when teenagers are driving, whether medication alters sleep initiation, and risk status for drug use.

You and your child's pediatrician will need to consider 3 elements when arriving at the best stimulant medication plan for your child: the type of stimulant medication, the dose, and the medication schedule. As we pointed out earlier, even though all of the commonly used stimulants can be equally successful at treating the symptoms of ADHD, it is not possible to predict which one or what dose will work best for a particular child.

Dosage

You may already be aware that the dosage of many medications, including antibiotics, cold medications, and other over-the-counter drugs, is determined by a child's weight. This is not the case with stimulant medications. Just as individual children respond differently to different stimulants, each child requires a different dosage that cannot be predicted in advance. The best dosage for a child with ADHD is the one that achieves the *best possible*

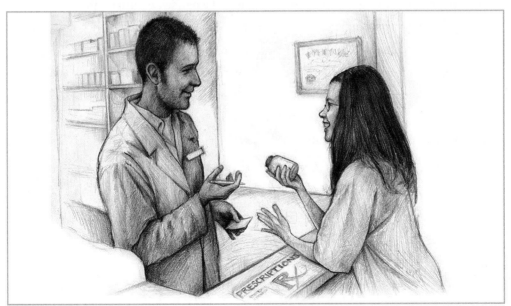

You can expect medication changes until you and your child's pediatrician arrive at the most effective medication and dosage for your child.

results without troublesome side effects—*not* the minimum dose that leads to any level of positive response (even though in the past this has been a fairly common practice among physicians). Because the dosage is determined by how well it works, and because it varies so widely among children, your child's pediatrician may need to adjust the dosage a number of times before finding the best level.

Your child's pediatrician may choose to start with a low dose, and progress through a series of dose increases, monitoring the results by feedback from you, your child, and her teacher. Often rating scales are given to parents and teachers to organize their observations concerning each dose. In general, you and your child should see your pediatrician in a face-to-face follow-up visit by the fourth week of medication use to review your child's response to the medication, including its effects on core symptoms, to monitor any side effects and check her blood pressure, pulse, and weight. Many physicians use rating scales like the Vanderbilt Scales (see Appendix) to organize parents' and teachers' observations. Also remember that you have already targeted specific behaviors that you hope to see improve with medication management. Ideally, your child's pediatrician will review these with you, and will also ask for teacher input regarding these targets in the form of a phone call or written report, perhaps supplemented with standardized behavior checklists. A good way to organize these reports is to set up a daily "report card" that can track teachers' observations about each target. The more objective these reports can be—for example, how many times in a half-hour period a child blurts out answers without raising her hand, or how many math problems were completed correctly in a 15-minute period—the better. These report cards can then be brought into the doctor's office for review.

Once your child's doctor has reviewed any changes in your child's core symptoms and target behaviors, the medication dose can be gradually adjusted upward until the best results are achieved. Again, your doctor may not stop increasing the dose when you first notice a positive result, but will likely continue to increase it until there is no further improvement. If a higher dose produces side effects or no further improvement, the dosage can be reduced. This gradual method of arriving at the proper dose (titration) can minimize some of the initial side effects that might have occurred if he had started with the higher dose from the beginning.

In some cases a particular stimulant will have little effect. If this is the case with your child, a second stimulant can be tried. If 2 or more stimulants fail to be effective (an uncommon occurrence), a review of her diagnosis may be in order—or a switch to an alternative medication plan that includes one of the non-stimulant medications described beginning on page 77.

Many parents become concerned that the frequent dosage and medication changes (particularly as the medication is being started) may mean that their child's pediatrician does not know what he is doing. On the contrary, the only way to know how effective stimulant medications will be is to try a given medication and review changes in an organized way over a period. So expect medication changes until you and your child's pediatrician arrive at the most effective medication and dosage for your child.

Medication Schedules

As is evident from the table, stimulants are available in short-acting (about 4 hours), intermediate-acting (6–8 hours), or extended-release (10–12 hours) forms, making the dosing schedule of your child's medication quite flexible. Your child need not be limited to only one form and, for example, you may choose to combine short-acting forms with intermediate-acting or extended-release forms to create a schedule that best suits her needs. Many children prefer to take a longer-acting preparation (8–12 hours) before leaving for school in the morning because this makes it unnecessary to take any medication at school (so that their classmates will not even know they are taking it). If your child has after-school activities that cause her to put off doing homework until after the longer-acting medication has worn off, she may want to use an additional short-acting dose at that later time. In this case, she could take an 8-hour dose in the morning before school and another 4-hour dose half an hour before beginning her homework in the evening. Some college students prefer 4-hour medications because they can schedule these doses for the times during the day when they most need the medication. Again, think of stimulants as helpful tools, like glasses—children can use them at the times of day when they need to focus or achieve other target outcomes, and may prefer not to use them at other times. Just as with glasses, continuous coverage throughout the entire day with minimal side effects would be ideal, and researchers are presently working toward this goal.

GENERAL CONSIDERATIONS WHEN TAKING STIMULANT MEDICATIONS

- In general, stimulants are considered quite safe and effective for the treatment of ADHD.

- Your child's growth in height should be monitored regularly. Children taking stimulants may have modest slowing of their rate of growth, especially if they are using high doses of stimulants and taking them over long periods.

- Your child's blood pressure and heart rate should be checked before and during treatment with stimulant medications. If your family history includes sudden unexplained death, let your pediatrician or primary care physician know. In that case, or if your child has a history of severe heart palpitations, exercise intolerance, fainting spells, or chest pain, your pediatrician will do a careful physical examination, may obtain an EKG, and may check with a cardiologist before starting stimulant medication.

- Your doctor will also likely consult with a cardiologist prior to starting medication if your child has a serious heart problem.

Some physicians suggest taking "medication holidays"—stopping medication on weekends, during summer vacation, or over other longer periods when they feel the child needs them less. These breaks may speak to a desire of parents or children to minimize the use of stimulants, but there is no reliable evidence indicating that the breaks are helpful or necessary from a medical point of view. In many cases, families find that continuing the medication schedule outside of school hours and school days helps family relationships by supporting better listening skills and helps the more hyperactive and impulsive child better enjoy social experiences such as scout meetings, church activities, and sports. (For more information on "medication holidays," see page 263.)

Side Effects

As discussed previously, the dose of your child's medication should be increased until optimal results are achieved without significant side effects. Only a small number of children who are introduced to stimulant medication in the systematic way we have described—and who follow their medication schedule consistently—will find side effects too intrusive. Any side effects that do occur are likely to be mild, and most can be relieved by adjusting the dose or schedule of medication or by switching to another stimulant. While each medication can potentially create side effects in some children, there is no way to predict which child will experience side effects with any one medication. One child may experience side effects on dextroamphetamine (Dexedrine) but not methylphenidate (Ritalin), for example, while another may report opposite results. Again, the only way to find out is to try a stimulant and monitor the results.

Side effects caused by stimulants tend to occur early in treatment and are generally mild. The most common side effects include a decreased appetite, stomachaches, headaches, difficulty falling asleep, jitteriness, and social withdrawal. Rarely, children who are overly sensitive to stimulants or on too high a dose can become overly focused and seem dull. Other less common side effects include dizziness, rebound effect (increased activity, irritability, or sadness for a short time as the medication wears off), and transient tics (repetitive eye blinking, shoulder shrugging, etc) most common when a new stimulant is first taken. In some children with Tourette disorder (Chapter 9) stimulants may make their tics worse.

Your child's pediatrician can help you manage most of these side effects through adjustments in dose amount or schedule, the use of alternative medication preparations, or occasionally by adding other medications. It is important to pay attention to the timing of side effects. For example, if your child seems irritable 4 hours after an intermediate-acting dose, this may suggest too high a dose of medication. If the irritability occurs 8 hours after an intermediate-acting medication, it may indicate a withdrawal or rebound effect.

EATING CHALLENGES

Decreased appetite and weight loss are common side effects of stimulant medication use. These typically occur early in treatment and are short-lived. If you find your child is losing weight or not eating enough consider the following tips listed below. Remember, your child's doctor can help you manage eating challenges so be sure to share any concerns.

- Encourage breakfast with calorie-dense foods. Examples: yogurt, eggs, fiber cereals, oatmeal.
- Provide nutritious after-school and bedtime snacks that are high in protein and in complex carbohydrates. Examples: whole-grain crackers and cheese, whole-grain pita with hummus, nutrition bars.
- Shift dinner to later in the evening when your child's medication has worn off. Or, allow "grazing" in the evening on healthy snacks as your child may be hungriest right before bed.

Adapted from: American Academy of Pediatrics. *ADHD—Caring for Children With ADHD: A Resource Toolkit for Clinicians.* Elk Grove Village, IL: American Academy of Pediatrics; 2005.

Special Circumstances: Preschool Children

A PARENT'S STORY
An Early Start to Treatment "I began seeing plausible signs of ADHD in my son when he was only 4 years old. He was very active, and overreacted to any bit of frustration in his life. When we tried to talk to him, he didn't seem interested in listening, and had trouble paying attention. He went to preschool, but was actually thrown out because he was so out of control." "His pediatrician diagnosed him as having ADHD, and although she told me and my husband that medication was an option that we could consider, I was very hesitant. I was nervous about side effects of medicines, and initially didn't want to go there. So with my doctor's guidance, we tried behavioral approaches like setting up reward systems. But none of them made much of a difference. We became more concerned that he was not able to follow directions at home, had great difficulty playing with friends, and didn't seem to be learning what other preschoolers usually know, even though we've always considered him really bright. We were also worried that he might not be able to handle a kindergarten classroom." "That's when we agreed to try medication. We tried low doses of methylphenidate. My son has been taking it for more than 4 months now, and we've seen a dramatic improvement in his behavior. He's back in preschool and, after a lot of struggling with this, we feel like we made the right decision." Diane, Los Angeles, CA

Behavioral management approaches should be tried before considering the use of stimulant mediations in preschool children. This is because

- Up to one-third of young children (aged 4–5) experience improvements in symptoms with behavior therapy alone.
- There are some concerns about whether the effects of stimulant medications on growth and other side effects may be heightened for preschool children.
- There is less information and experience about the effects of stimulant medication between the ages of 4 and 5 years than for older children.

Many 4- and 5-year-olds with ADHD may still require medication to achieve maximum improvement. The decision to consider using stimulant medication at this age depends in part on how severely a child's symptoms of ADHD are interfering with his development and other aspects of his life such as safety risks, consequences for school, and limitations on social participation.

Although dextroamphetamine is the only medication approved for children younger than 6, there is very limited information on this drug in children this young. Most of the evidence about the safety and positive effects of treating preschool children with stimulant medications has been limited to methylphenidate. There is a growing body of evidence that methylphenidate is safe and efficacious in preschool-aged children; however, its use in preschool-aged children remains an "off-label" use of the medication, as it is not FDA approved for children younger than 6. If preschoolers do not experience adequate symptom improvement with behavioral therapy, medication can be prescribed. Preschool-aged children are generally started at a lower dose, and medication doses are increased in smaller increments. Maximum doses have not been adequately studied.

Monitoring the Results

When stimulants are tried in the systematic way described in this chapter, at least 80% of children will respond well to one of them. The key word here is "systematic." The medication must be initially prescribed according to a reliable plan. After the initial dose has been established, adjustments can be made in response to frequent, regular feedback provided by you, your child, *and her teachers.* To avoid the natural tendency to believe a method is working just because it is being used, your child's pediatrician should

- Regularly see your child and ask her and you about her medication.
- Regularly ask you specific questions about behavior and academic performance.
- Help you develop a tool like home and school "report cards" (see the box on page 74) to measure progress relating to the target outcomes you have selected.
- Ask your child's teacher structured questions or ask him to complete structured behavioral and performance rating scales, rather than simply asking you if your child is "doing better." Systematic teacher input is especially important when starting medication or changing the dose.

DAILY SCHOOL-HOME REPORT CARDS

Daily report cards can help provide immediate feedback on your child's behavior. This feedback can be used to help you and your child's pediatrician decide if your target goals are being met and if medication adjustments might be helpful. Some typical target areas include

- Academic productivity
- Following classroom rules
- Peer relationships
- Teacher relationships
- Behavior outside the classroom
- Time-out behavior
- Responsibility for belongings
- Homework

After picking the most appropriate general target areas for your child, as you read in Chapter 2, you will need to describe representative behaviors in detail. For example, if "behavior outside the classroom" is a major problem, your target behavior list might include items like

- Follows the rules at lunch and in the hallway with 4 or fewer violations per week
- Walks in line appropriately (appropriate behavior needs to be defined and agreed on)
- Follows the rules on the bus with 2 or fewer violations per week
- Needs 2 or fewer warnings for exhibiting inappropriate table manners in the lunchroom per week (eg, playing with food, throwing trash on the floor)
- Changes into gym clothes within 6 minutes

Note that these items are all carefully defined and countable. This makes it easier to track progress. The number of allowable violations listed should also be realistic enough that the goals can be achieved. You will read more about school-home report cards in Chapter 7.

Adapted with permission from: William E. Pelham Jr, PhD. School-Home Daily Report Card packet available for downloading at no cost at http://ccf.buffalo.edu. Also see American Academy of Pediatrics. *ADHD: Caring for Children With ADHD: A Resource Toolkit for Clinicians.* Elk Grove Village, IL: American Academy of Pediatrics; 2005.

Structured questions, reports, charts, and rating scales from teachers can also measure (in numeric terms wherever possible) any improvement in your child's treatment targets, such as classroom productivity, on-task behavior, and other function-related goals. Because many of the better rating scales your child's pediatrician will be familiar with have been used on a broad sample of hundreds of children the same age as yours, they will place your child's performance in the context of her peers and classmates. By continuing to assess and measure selected targets in a consistent way, you can also compare your child's performance with how she was doing 2, 6, or 12 months ago.

As you begin to review your child's progress, keep in mind that children respond at different rates in different target areas, and that not all of the goals that you set for your child can be turned into targets that are medication-sensitive. Almost everyone who is hyperactive improves rapidly on some dose of stimulant medication. But, for example, if inattention has led to falling behind in reading, it may take several weeks or months to see improvement. However, if the reading lag is due to a learning disability (see Chapter 7) rather than poor attention while learning, it will not be expected to respond to medication management and will need additional educational interventions.

As always, your focus should remain much more on improvements in your child's ability to function in the previously identified target areas—whenever possible, assessing behaviors that can be counted and measured—rather than on general impressions about improvement in "his ADHD." When attending follow-up visits with your child's doctor, come prepared with specific (and, if possible, countable) examples of changes in the target areas you are measuring. If you have been using school-home report cards, you should chart them. You can also ask your child's teachers to prepare a narrative report of your child's progress since your last visit, or fill out any specific rating scales suggested by your child's pediatrician that could be used for making decisions about the medication management plan. During your visit, these materials should be reviewed before determining whether any changes need to be made in the dose, scheduling, or type of stimulant medication. The more systematically and frequently feedback from home and school is obtained at follow-up visits, the greater improvement your child is likely to experience.

One major reason for frequent follow-up visits is to make certain that your child's medication dose is optimal. In the large ADHD treatment study (the Multimodal Treatment Study of Children with Attention Deficit Hyperactivity Disorder [MTA]) described in Chapter 3 and on page 50, special care was taken to find an optimal dose of medication according to preset guidelines during the first few weeks of treatment. These optimal doses were higher on average than among children who were not on the study medication management guidelines but being treated by the individual plans of their own physicians. In addition, the dosage in the study guidelines spanned the school day as well as the early evening, as opposed to the common practice of prescribing just enough medication to cover the school day. Once treatment began, children and families in the study met with their physician for half an hour each month to discuss concerns and review the teacher's monthly report. During these sessions a great deal of parent and child education was carried out. Changes in the child's treatment were then made, if necessary, in response to feedback from parents and schoolteachers. If the child experienced difficulties, the physician adjusted the medication, and these adjustments occurred frequently. In contrast, the children with ADHD being treated by their own physicians in the community generally met with them only once or twice a year, had shorter and less comprehensive visits, were on lower doses of stimulant medication, and had teachers who were not as consistently involved in the treatment process.

As was pointed out in Chapter 3, about 60% of children with ADHD who received this optimal dose of medication with frequent and regular doctor visits and careful monitoring by parents and teachers were rated by teachers as indistinguishable in many areas from their peers without ADHD. This was even more enhanced with a combined medication and behavior approach. However, only about 25% of children being treated for ADHD by their own physicians (and most of the time the treatments included medication) were so rated. Experts feel that this may be due, to a large extent, to not following the kind of careful and organized approaches discussed previously.

Of course you live in the real world, not under the ideal conditions of a study. Monthly visits are impractical. But by using the principles used in the MTA study—using a medication dose that causes the most improvement (rather than the lowest possible dose), making sure that homework time is also covered by medication, setting up reasonably frequent and highly structured follow-up visits, etc—you can achieve the best evidence-based medication regulation possible for your child.

If your child has tried 2 or 3 stimulants and none have helped, or if your child had side effects that could not be controlled, another type of medication may be an option. Stimulants also may not be an option for children who are taking certain other medications or who have certain medical conditions. In these situations, ask your child's pediatrician for advice and refer to the information on non-stimulants below.

Costs of stimulant medication can vary widely, and paying for prescriptions can be a challenge, whether one has health insurance or not. Wholesale prices of different preparations of the same FDA-approved medication for ADHD can also differ significantly. If you find yourself unable to afford the cost of medications, contact your state's pharmacy assistance program to see if you are eligible for assistance. For further details, visit the National Resource Center on ADHD at www.help4adhd.org.

What Other Types of Medications Are Available?

Proven alternate choices to stimulant medications include atomoxetine, guanfacine XR, and bupropion. Because they have not been studied as rigorously or used as much as stimulants, most of these medications are considered second-line (second-choice) treatments. Some non-stimulants may be appropriate for children who have been diagnosed with ADHD and certain coexisting conditions—such as ADHD with accompanying tic disorders (such as Tourette disorder)—because they can in some cases treat both conditions simultaneously.

Atomoxetine

Atomoxetine (Strattera) is a non-stimulant approved by the FDA for the treatment of ADHD. It is in the class of medications known as selective norepinephrine reuptake inhibitors. Because atomoxetine does not seem to have a potential for abuse, it is not classified as a controlled substance. At the same time, because atomoxetine is a newer medication, the evidence supporting its use is more limited than for stimulants. Atomoxetine, unlike stimulants, is active around the clock. However, atomoxetine has been found to be only about two-thirds as effective as stimulant medications. After starting atomoxetine it may take up to 6 weeks before it reaches its maximum effectiveness. Atomoxetine has a warning on it that it may, in a very small number of cases, have some potential for causing suicidal thoughts in the first few weeks of treatment. On the other hand, atomoxetine may be helpful in the treatment of children who have both ADHD and anxiety. Side effects are generally mild but can include decreased appetite, upset stomach, nausea or vomiting, tiredness, problems sleeping, and dizziness. Jaundice is mentioned in a warning on the medication, but is extremely rare. Taking atomoxetine with food can help avoid nausea and stomachaches. Atomoxetine should be used in lower doses in children also taking certain antidepressants like fluoxetine (Prozac) or paroxetine (Paxil), because it can raise the atomoxetine levels in the bloodstream.

Atomoxetine is now considered an option for first-line therapy for ADHD, and is the first non-stimulant to fall into the first-line category. Parents concerned about the possibility that stimulants may be used for substance abuse may choose atomoxetine as the first-line agent for their child. It is often used for children who have had unsuccessful trials of stimulants.

Long-Acting Guanfacine and Other Alpha Agonists

Long-acting guanfacine (Intuniv) is in the group of medications known as alpha agonists. These medications were developed for the treatment of high blood pressure but have also been used to treat children with ADHD who have tics, sleep problems, and/or aggression. It has recently been approved by the FDA for the treatment of children with ADHD. Long-acting guanfacine is a pill, but it cannot be crushed, chewed, or broken and must be swallowed whole. Like atomoxetine, it is not a controlled substance. It does not cause much appetite suppression, so may be a good choice for children who lost a significant amount of weight when taking a stimulant. Side effects can include sleepiness, headaches, fatigue, stomachaches, nausea, lethargy, dizziness, irritability, decreased blood pressure, and decreased appetite. Although sleepiness occurs in a large number of children when children start taking long-acting guanfacine, it seems to get better as they continue to take it. It may take 3 to 4 weeks to see medication benefit. Two other shorter-acting alpha agonists are available for use, but not approved by the FDA for ADHD. These are clonidine (Catapres) and short-acting guanfacine (Tenex). These can be used as adjunctive medications, or if FDA-approved medications are not helpful. If no FDA-approved medication has been found helpful for your child, you should also consider whether ADHD is the correct diagnosis, and whether additional coexisting conditions (Chapter 9) might be present. The alpha agonists can be used to treat tics, and because about half of children who have a tic disorder called Tourette disorder (Chapter 9) also have ADHD, they may be useful in this context.

Bupropion

Bupropion is a unique type of antidepressant that has been less frequently studied as a treatment for ADHD. It is also not FDA approved for ADHD. Some research that has been done indicates that bupropion is effective in reducing ADHD symptoms in some children, but it seems to have less effect than stimulants or atomoxetine. Its use in ADHD is not widespread. The side effects, though usually minimal, can include irritability, decreased appetite, insomnia, and a worsening of existing tics. It is important to note that at higher doses, bupropion may make some individuals more prone to seizures, so it should be used cautiously in children who have seizure disorders.

NON-STIMULANT MEDICATIONS USED FOR ADHD

Generic Class (Brand Name)	Daily Dosage	Prescribing Schedule
ATOMOXETINE (Strattera)	Once a day to twice a day	0.5 mg/kg per day increasing to 1.4 mg/kg per day
GUANFACINE Long-acting (Intuniv) Short-acting (Tenex)	1–4 mg daily 1–2 mg 2 to 3 times daily	Start at lower doses
CLONIDINE Oral tablets Film patches	0.1–0.3 mg 2 to 3 times daily 0.1–0.3 mg patch daily	Start at lower doses
BUPROPION Short-acting (Wellbutrin) Intermediate (Wellbutrin SR) Long-acting (Wellbutrin XL)	3 times daily, no single dose >150 mg 2 times daily, no single dose >150 mg Once daily (twice if single dose >150 mg)	150–300 mg per day 150–300 mg per day 150–300 mg per day

How Can I Talk to My Child About Medication?

If medication issues seem complex and sometimes confusing to parents of children with ADHD, they can be even more so to the children themselves. Your child may strongly resist the idea of sticking to a regular schedule of medication—because she fears that this will remind her on a daily basis that she is not "normal" or that other children will tease her, because she resents the intrusion in her everyday routine, because she is afraid of the consequences of taking any medication, or because she strongly wishes to control her own behavior.

The more information you can give your child about medications, the more actively and productively she can participate in her own treatment decisions. In fact, while on a medication she should be better able to accurately evaluate her own behavior and performance. Parents sometimes worry that their child will begin to attribute her successes to the medication rather than to herself but, in fact, children on medication most often cite their own efforts or abilities (not the medication) as the explanation for their success. All of this is important because children's active participation in their own treatment plans leads to better treatment results. Sometimes she may not notice any changes in herself, but will notice that she gets into less trouble or completes more of her work.

To some degree (depending on her age and level of comprehension) your child will need to know what stimulants are, what effects they are likely to have, how long most children continue to take them, how doses and schedules can vary, and how the treatment process is likely to proceed. Medications should be discussed as tools that can be used effectively or ineffectively to achieve behavior or learning goals. As you and your child's doctors explain these issues, encourage your child to ask questions, voice her fears and concerns, and incorporate her ideas into the medication treatment plan. Your child's desire to address her problems "on her own" may not be an option, but respecting her input and discussing the medication with her is important.

If your child is upset or worried about other children making fun of her, remind her that long-lasting stimulants can make it unnecessary for her to take the medication at school. (Your own efforts to educate her about medication will help bolster her confidence as well, making her less vulnerable to this type of teasing.) Especially if she complains about having to take pills every day, allow her to provide input regarding her dosage regimen. By high school, depending on study habits and extracurricular activities, her medication plan may need to change again. For example, the 12-hour dose from 7:00 am to 7:00 pm that worked well in junior high school may need to be reconsidered if her homework now usually gets done between 7:00 pm and 11:00 pm.

As your child begins the process of taking medication, first and foremost, listen carefully to her. If she reports that she "feels different," consider whether she is reporting side effects or just describing the hoped-for positive effects of the medication. Remind her (and yourself) that the goal is to preserve all of her positive personality traits, help her focus and allow her mental time to think before doing—so that she can think about her choices and pick the best one.

In general, helping your child become as knowledgeable as possible about the effects and side effects of medications should lead to greater engagement in her own treatment. One of the ways in which she can maximize the potential of her prescribed medication is to monitor her own responses to it and report them to the other members of her treatment team. She should be sufficiently aware of possible side effects so she can report them to the treatment team if and when they occur. She should also report any positive effects and actively participate in at least part of all meetings where her treatment is discussed. Your child's pediatrician should take the time to explain to her how any changes in her functioning have come about—particularly which are the result of the medication versus which are due to her own efforts.

Your child should also understand the limitations of medication—that while medication can help with the core symptoms of ADHD, she will need to use this advantage to actively improve her functioning in her target areas. With consistent effort and education she can learn to use her medication to help her overcome social, academic, and behavioral challenges. But if she leaves all the work to the medication, she will see fewer positive results.

Many new issues can arise during the teenage years. As your child approaches adolescence, it will be appropriate to transfer to her as much of the responsibility for her medication regimen as she is able to responsibly handle. For example, a teenager may actually begin to dislike the feelings that a particular medication creates so a reconsideration of the dose or specific medication may be a reasonable solution. A teenager who takes an active part in her treatment plan is likely to consider these options, whereas one who is not involved with the treatment plan may decide to just stop taking the medication. The more empowered a teenager feels in her own treatment the more likely she is to be an active participant. Teenagers may have a particularly hard time accepting the idea of taking medications due to their age-appropriate desire for independence, resistance to adult direction, and need to conform to their peers. The best way to deal with your teenager's new attitudes toward medications is to listen even more openly to her opinions and feelings on the issue and to allow her as much control of her treatment as possible. Because this is a time developmentally when youths may begin to experiment with drugs (including stimulants), your teenager may realize that the medications can have a "street value." This issue warrants a serious discussion. Teenagers do not want to stand out or be different, and they may begin to question whether they still need to take medications. Teenagers who "own" their own problems, successes, and treatment plan by this age will do much better with continuing their treatment. At times it may be helpful to have a period off of medication with structured teacher feedback to demonstrate to your teenager the significant differences that medications can make.

Your teenager needs to be involved in all areas of decision-making related to her medication management. As an adult, she will need to be able to routinely manage her own medication and other issues related to ADHD. Her desire to begin practicing self-management now is a healthy sign of growth, and should be encouraged with your careful attention and guidance. The bottom line here is that the more empowered your teenager feels in her own treatment process at all stages of development, the more likely she is to live up to her responsibilities—and the more effective her treatment plan will be.

Making the Most of Medication

It is important to remember that medication is only one component of your child's treatment, but can provide a powerful springboard from which your child can begin to master the challenges of ADHD. While it can be difficult at first to understand and properly use any type of medication, you and your child will soon grow comfortable with the routines and considerations that can maximize its benefits. You, your child, and her teachers must actively monitor its effects and discuss them with her pediatrician. To enjoy maximum success, effective parenting techniques and teaching and self-management tools (see chapters 5 and 6) will also need to be used where appropriate. Treatment plans that include medication and effective behavior therapy may result in lower doses of medication necessary to achieve academic, behavioral, and social goals.

Over time, you will find that active monitoring of and participating in your child's treatment can be extremely rewarding for you and your child as you watch her day-to-day functioning, performance, and self-esteem improve. In the meantime, as you become acquainted with the process of using medications, consider sharing your new experiences with other families in your situation. Your local support group for children with ADHD and their parents can provide you with validation and practical advice during this challenging time. As you will discover, many families have been where you find yourselves today—and most will tell you how glad they are that they informed themselves about this type of treatment as they took action regarding their child's future.

Q & A

Q: *I've noticed that, especially on days when my son hasn't had a lot of sleep or he's under some kind of stress, he tends to lose control of his behavior in extreme ways toward the end of his dosage. Any disruption in his life—a change of plans or a "time out"—will cause him to go into a tantrum or lash out against family members. Is this a side effect of the medication, and is there any way to avoid it?*

A: Some children do experience the kind of "behavioral rebound" effect you describe—most often in the early days of medication use as they are adjusting to the medication. It is important to report these symptoms to your child's physician who prescribed the medication, and to monitor the effects from day to day and over time. In most cases, this rebound effect lasts for only a short period right around the time that the medication is wearing off. It also typically becomes much less of a problem within a period of several days after starting a particular medication or changing a dose. If rebound remains a problem, it can usually be helped by changing the time of medication administration, changing the medication preparation to a longer-acting form, or adding a small dosing about 30 minutes prior to the onset of rebound symptoms. If these measures do not help, then an alternative medication should be considered. Sleep deprivation can add to difficulties.

Q: *My 14-year-old daughter began taking stimulants for her ADHD 6 months ago. Though we were all hesitant at first to try medication, the results were so clearly positive when she did try it that we had no problem continuing. Lately, though, my daughter has begun "forgetting" to take her pill in the morning. The more we remind her, the more resistant she gets. Her typical response is, "OK, Mom, I'll take it! Do you think I forgot for a minute that I have ADHD?" So far, she hasn't missed her medication more than one or two days in a row, but we fear these lapses may grow more frequent if we don't figure out why they're happening. Is this kind of resistance common with most kids with ADHD?*

A: Medication continues to carry with it a stigma that many children with ADHD—particularly early adolescents—feel acutely as they try to fit in with their peer group in the neighborhood and at school. In addition, adolescents with ADHD must negotiate the same process of seeking independence from parents that all teenagers do. Your daughter's resistance to taking medication despite its obvious benefits is not unusual, though it is an issue that needs to be addressed. While there is no one-size-fits-all solution to your situation, you should work with your daughter and the rest of your treatment team toward a positive approach. This may involve allowing her more control of the medication process—letting her make decisions about when and where she takes the medication—as well as control over the dosage schedule. Because she is first starting medication in her teenage years, it is important that she had buy-in to the initial trial of medication and that it was carried out in a manner that clearly demonstrated to her that the medication had a clear, positive effect. It is also important that she remain as informed as possible about the medication and all aspects of her medication management.

Chapter 5

Managing ADHD at Home

A number of specific home measures and parenting techniques have been shown to significantly improve the functioning of many children with attention-deficit/hyperactivity disorder (ADHD). When properly implemented and consistently applied, these approaches may not only help reshape your child's behavior at home and in public, but also decrease tension, strengthen family relationships, improve school performance, and lead to an increase in your child's self-esteem. Introducing and maintaining new routines and styles of interaction are never easy, but it is worth the effort to observe for yourself that children with ADHD can and do learn, adapt, and succeed.

Medication management and behavior therapy are the most proven, evidence-based mainstays of treatments for ADHD. They can measurably improve the lives of many children with ADHD and their families. There are also many other helpful general approaches to parenting and to your child's everyday life at home that can increase the positive effects achieved through these forms of treatment, create a supportive and structured home environment, foster positive family relationships, and bolster your child's self-esteem. This chapter will review these measures.

In this chapter, you will learn how to

- Help your child focus on his strengths rather than directing attention to his disabilities.
- Simplify, organize, and structure his home environment to help him succeed.
- Monitor your child's daily routines and rhythms and use this knowledge to help him become better regulated.
- Facilitate better communication with your child and within the family.
- Organize your own life in ways that will allow you to manage your family's challenges and have time for yourself.
- Help your child establish and maintain new, rewarding relationships.

Focusing on Strengths

All children, whether or not they have ADHD, do best when their parents build on their strengths. By identifying and nurturing your own child's special abilities and talents, you can encourage the self-esteem, confidence, and competence necessary for him to succeed in life despite the obstacles that stand in his way. These strengths might include being dedicated, fast on his feet, seeing things that others do not, creative thinking, and family oriented, as well as many other talents that will serve him well throughout childhood, adolescence, and his adult life.

One of the best ways to help your child focus on what he can do, rather than what he cannot, is to help him experience as many concrete successes as possible. The more he sees what he can accomplish in his world, the more optimistic and confident he is likely to feel. Instruction in any of your child's evolving interests—sports, art, computers, woodworking, music, martial arts, or any other area—can lay the groundwork for such achievement, especially when combined with your praise for his efforts as well as his successes. If your child's interests are not clear, help him discover and define some by actively finding areas where he can succeed. Talking with your child and supporting what he most enjoys and is best at may help him start to think about who he is and what he can do instead of who or what he is not.

The Primary Need for Your Child to Be a Child

The richness of childhood includes being allowed to play, explore, test, make mistakes as well as good choices, be oppositional as well as well behaved, etc. Part of allowing developmentally appropriate growth in children is to engage in daily activity without being constantly corrected. You are encouraged to keep this in mind as you seek help and readjust the roles of all family members. For example, few experts would disagree with limiting television and video game time. There is even some evidence that children with ADHD clock more hours of video watching and video games than other children. Excessive video viewing in early childhood may be associated with a higher risk for developing ADHD. There is also evidence that excessive media consumption, especially computer game playing, can impair sleep patterns and verbal cognitive performance in children. A reasonable approach to these issues is to limit screen time, and let this time be dependent on completing household tasks and homework. On the other hand, knowledge of appropriate television shows and video games is an important aspect of many children's social life and ability to make friends and share interests. All parents need to constantly walk this fine line. It may be tempting for parents with children with ADHD to become overly cautions or restrictive, or rule-bound because of good advice (as below). A good question to ask for any plan that you consider adopting is "How does it encourage and foster healthy development as well as relationships with family members?"

Simplifying, Organizing, and Structuring the Home Environment

You will find that your child's ability to progress in nearly all areas of self-management and social interaction increases when his environment is organized and structured to meet his unique needs. If your child is physically impulsive or accident-prone, take the time to unclutter and safety-proof your home. Some children with ADHD may benefit from an orderly physical environment with a place for each object, while keeping the environment (eg, your child's room) organized may be a hopeless task for others. Try helping your child organize his room at a level he can manage.

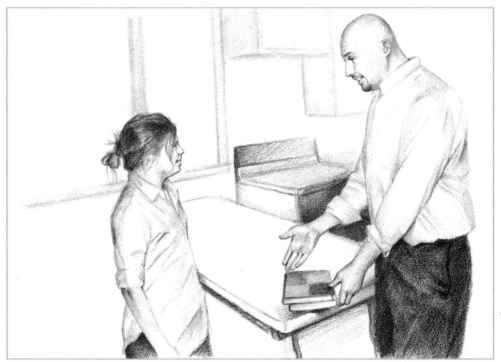

If your child has specific and logical places to keep her schoolwork, toys, and clothes, she is less likely to lose them.

Daily routines are an absolute necessity for many children with ADHD. Consistent limit-setting with predictable consequences, along with limited choices (not "What do you want to eat?" but "Do you want an apple or a boiled egg?"), also make your child's world more manageable and help him meet his goals. Written lists of chores or other daily tasks are especially useful in helping your child keep track of what he needs to do, and is an excellent habit for him to carry into adolescence and adulthood.

When considering how to structure your child's day-to-day experiences, it may help to picture your growing child as a construction project in progress. The limits, lists, routines, and other measures you are putting in place today are like scaffolding that will provide the necessary support as he develops fully. As he turns these routines into daily habits and becomes more self-directed, some of these supports can be gradually removed while his underlying functioning remains well in place. (You may no longer have to create homework checklists with him, for example, because he has learned to make them himself.) Far from "babying" your child, helping to structure and organize his world allows him to add to his competencies and experience many more small triumphs, increasing his self-esteem.

Just as you have observed that your child may feel less overwhelmed when his home life is well organized, so you may find that organizing your own family life as thoroughly as possible will help you feel calmer and more in control. (This is even more likely to be the case, of course, if you have ADHD.) With the number of medical visits, teachers' conferences, and treatment reviews necessary to maintain your child's well-being and continued progress, a family calendar including all scheduled activities can be an essential for many families. Daily lists of tasks to perform and errands to run will help you stay organized just as they help your child. Many parents find it worthwhile to devote a private 10 minutes to half an hour before the kids get up in the morning to "regroup"—thinking about everything that must be accomplished that day and arranging tasks in order of priority. Make sure that any plan is realistic and not overwhelming.

TIPS FOR STRUCTURING YOUR CHILD'S HOME ENVIRONMENT

Remember that the success of rules and strategies within your home is influenced by the quality of the relationship that you have with your child and/or adolescent.

- **Keep your child on a daily schedule.** Try to keep the time that your child wakes up, eats, bathes, leaves for school, and goes to sleep about the same each day.
  - Be prepared for transitions and shifts in routines or projects.
  - Try to give time warnings when an activity or event is going to be taking place. Give 15-, 10-, and 5-minute warnings for changes in activity. Examples are coming to dinner, doing homework, turning off the television set, bedtime, etc.
  - Schedule unconditional "fun" time regularly.

- **Cut down on distractions.** Identify the things that distract your child the most at important times (like during homework), but do not jump to conclusions—the distractions for each child are different. As you identify them, eliminate them one by one.

- **Develop a homework plan with your child.**
  - Create a special homework space with your child and stock it with supplies for projects and homework.
  - Keep in mind, some children like having a mini office set up. Others need to be close to mom or dad.
  - Use a homework incentive chart with rewards.
  - Have a second set of schoolbooks at home.
  - Divide homework into small working parts with breaks.
  - Use special timers to keep your child on track.
  - Share homework detail with other family members.
  - Save a spot near the door for the school backpack so your child can grab it on the way out the door (place a hook by the back door to hang it up after homework).

- **Organize your house.** If your child has specific and logical places to keep his schoolwork, toys, and clothes, he is less likely to lose them.
  - Develop "house rules," monitor daily, and reward for compliance of rules. (Pick one house rule weekly to review and discuss as a family.)
  - Provide a safe space in the home for active play.

TIPS FOR STRUCTURING YOUR CHILD'S HOME ENVIRONMENT (CONTINUED)

- **Use charts and checklists.** These written reminders can help your child track his progress with chores or homework. Keep instructions brief. Offer frequent, friendly reminders to check his list and make sure each task has been completed.
  - Implement the use of a school-home tracker. (A tracker is a checklist of things needed each day to take to school and a checklist of things needed to bring home from school.)
  - Post a checklist by the morning exit door to the school bus listing the things that need to go to school, such as backpack, shoes, coat, gloves, and lunch box.
  - Focus on the effort your child made to do their work and chores, not just the completion of the task.

- **Limit choices.** Help your child learn to make good decisions by giving him only 2 or 3 options at a time.
  - **Foster "best outcomes" by creating and encouraging a sense of resiliency and participation.**
    o Validate your child's positive plans even if you feel some things need to be done differently.
    o Express empathy for concerns and problems.
    o Include your teenager in the decision-making process and problem-solving issues.
    o Encourage involvement in family activity planning and outings.
    o Provide sincere praise, even for the small things.

- **Set small, reachable goals.** Aim for systematic step-by-step progress rather than instant results. Be sure that your child understands that he can succeed best by taking small steps and slowly building on those successes.
  - **Keep the plan child-centered.** Even though the plan may work well for you, make sure that it works for your child or it will turn out to be ineffective.

Daily Routines and Rhythms

As the parent of a child with ADHD, you may already be aware of certain times of day that are more difficult than others. If your child has begun taking a stimulant medication, you may notice fluctuations in his attention and behavioral control throughout the day as each dose of medication begins to take effect, works well, and then wears off. With stimulant medications, effects such as behavioral rebound (a short period of irritability or moodiness as the medication is wearing off in about 4, 8, or 12 hours [see Chapter 4]) may lead to difficulties at around dinnertime or bedtime that had not generally occurred before. You can help your child adjust to these changes by observing how and when his emotions and behavior tend to fluctuate each day and arranging his schedule as much as possible to accommodate these ups and downs. If you know, for example, that he is usually somewhat unsettled and irritable for a half an hour after his arrival home from school, schedule his homework for after that time. If his medication suppresses his appetite at certain times during the day, schedule meals to avoid these periods. Take special care to prepare him for transitions between activities because these are likely to be especially difficult times for him.

Another issue to consider is the way a specific length of time can sometimes feel to a child with ADHD. For a child who struggles with managing his behavior or retaining focus for more than a few minutes at a time, tedious, repetitive, or boring activities can seem extra long and soon become absolutely unbearable. Forcing your child to participate in such an activity (requiring him to sit still for long periods while you chat with a friend, introducing him to clubs or groups that involve little physical action and too much downtime, expecting him to pick up all the toys at once in a disorderly room) will probably only lead to failure and the probability of subsequent punishment and/or lower self-esteem. Even fun activities can be strenuous in the same way. For example, baseball, which includes long periods of inactivity while on the field, may not be as good an activity for children with ADHD as soccer, which has a much faster and continuous pace. By avoiding such situations or breaking up activities (including homework) into short chunks of time, you can help your child experience success as he struggles to manage his responses. It may also help to let your child know ahead of time how long a particular activity will last, and even to place a timer in view to help his awareness of how much time has passed. If he knows he has already been working on his homework or practicing the piano for more than half the allotted time, he may be able (with your support and coaching) to continue to the end.

THE FIRST HOUR OF THE DAY

The morning routine can be a daunting task for all parents and children. Pressures to get to school and work can feel overwhelming at times. For a child with ADHD, getting the day started can be especially challenging. To ease the stress on your child, create a consistent and predictable schedule for rising and set up a manageable routine. It may help to put specific steps in writing or pictures keeping the tasks clear and brief. For example, alarm rings ➪wash face ➪get dressed (with clothes laid out the night before) ➪eat breakfast ➪take medication ➪brush teeth.

Remember to give immediate praise and feedback when your child accomplishes tasks of the "morning routine." This will help motivate your child to succeed and encourage independence.

If your child takes medication, your doctor may recommend waking your child up 30 to 45 minutes before the usual wake time to give medication and then let your child "rest" in bed for the next 30 minutes. This rest period allows the medication to begin working so that your child can be better able to participate in the morning routine.

TIPS FOR MANAGING SLEEP PROBLEMS

Many children with ADHD have trouble getting to sleep at night, whether or not they take medication. Good bedtime habits (sleep hygiene) can be a key to good sleep. These include

- Establish bedtime routines such as a warning that bedtime is in 15 minutes; a regular and routine order of toileting, brushing teeth, getting into pajamas, a short bedtime story or other interaction with parent.
- Fall asleep with lights off and no television or music.
- Always falling asleep in their own bed with parents out of the room can play a significant role in children being able to sleep through the night without disrupted sleep.

Medication Effects May Vary

- Some children fall asleep more easily if the medication has "worn off" by bedtime. Other children may have a more difficult time, and an evening dose of medication can help.
- Sometimes different preparations of stimulant medication can have different effects on sleep initiation in a given child, and a medication switch may help.
- Natural sleep aides like melatonin (3 mg 1–2 hours before bedtime) may be of considerable help, but always check with your child's doctor before using preparations, even if they are over-the-counter.
- Other medications are sometimes prescribed by physicians if the above measures are not successful and sleep issues are still interfering with day-to-day functioning.

Adapted from: American Academy of Pediatrics. ADHD—Caring for Children With ADHD: A Resource Toolkit for Clinicians. Elk Grove Village, IL: American Academy of Pediatrics; 2005.

Optimizing and Facilitating Communication

Children with ADHD frequently experience difficulty participating in elements of sustained and focused day-to-day conversation. But adapting your own style of communication to your child's needs can help him maintain a connection. When necessary, pause to get your child's attention (call his name before giving a command), maintain eye contact, and perhaps have him repeat back or explain what you have told him to be sure he has heard and understands. This approach works well not only when issuing commands but also when beginning any sort of conversation with your child. If he tends to interrupt, help him out by keeping your sentences brief and focusing only on what needs to be said. Avoid interrupting him frequently because he may not be able to stay engaged in this type of interaction. If you sense that his attention is wandering, touch his arm, take his hand, or otherwise make physical contact. Some parents find that conversation flows more smoothly if they are also involved in a physical activity with their child, such as washing dishes or making dinner. Finally, if you are telling your child something that you want him to remember, write it down in simple terms or encourage him to write it down himself. Introducing concepts such as "consequences," "rewards," and "positive and negative behavior" into the family vocabulary can go a long way toward clarifying communications. Where you might have previously instructed your child to "Go to your room!" following an unacceptable behavior, you can now inform him that his behavior has led to a "time-out"—and by the time you give this command, he will know the exact rules that apply to this term. Specific behavior therapy language strategies, such as when/then statements ("When you finish your homework, then you can go play baseball.") may also prove useful when interacting with all of your children and can improve communication and morale in the family as a whole.

Educating, Reframing, and Demystifying

Children with ADHD face a daily struggle with adult disapproval and other negative interactions that result from their behavioral and social difficulties. Such frequent negativity can easily lead to a loss of confidence and low self-esteem that, if left unaddressed, can result in even more self-defeating behavior. Designing an effective treatment plan is one way to prevent this negative cycle from occurring with your child because it is likely to lead to more positive feedback and better self-control. You can further increase your child's chances for improvement by taking the following steps:

- **Educate** your child about ADHD and how to manage it.
- **Reframe** any negative attitudes or assumptions and reshape the responses that have developed as a result of these attitudes and assumptions.
- **Demystify** the treatment process and clear up any misunderstandings.

The more fully a child with ADHD can begin to understand and "take ownership" of his own challenges, the more committed he is likely to be to treatment, the more successful he may become at self-management, and the higher his self-esteem is likely to be. Thus *educating* your child about the nature of ADHD is a critical part of successful treatment at every stage of development. From very early on, you and your child's pediatrician can begin talking with your child about the nature of ADHD, what it is and what it is not, and how he can learn to manage it. As he grows older, his pediatrician or other health care professional can meet with him alone so that he can feel free to seek any information he needs to become the most active participant in his own care plan. He may also benefit a great deal from your efforts to provide him with developmentally appropriate books about ADHD and responsible Web sites (see the Resources section on page 311) that provide updated information on ADHD and related disorders. Support groups for children and families with ADHD are another source of valuable information as well as an emotional resource. By his teenage years, your child should have had the opportunity to build up an informed knowledge base on which to rely when he (with your support) is making decisions about treatment, social and academic pursuits, plans for the future, and so on. Taking control of his own life in this way can be enormously empowering for a child who has struggled with ADHD and can make all the difference in how he views his life and academic, professional, and personal potential.

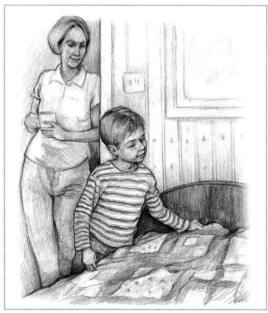

Focus on the effort your child made to do a chore, not just completion of the task.

As your child grows, keep in mind that he may forget or misinterpret some of what he is told about the nature of ADHD. To minimize his confusion, make sure that you and his pediatrician talk with him regularly and repeatedly about ADHD (not just at the first meeting) and ask him to repeat back to you what he understands, listening carefully to his interpretations of what he has learned. Always keep these discussions positive, simple and brief enough for him to participate fully. The clearer he is about who he is and where he stands in relation to ADHD, the more competence and confidence he will have in managing his challenges.

Because discouragement is a constant danger for children who face such frequent obstacles, be prepared to confront your child's negative ideas and statements, and help him reframe them in positive ways. "Everyone has attention problems from time to time. I just have them so often that they interfere with my best functioning—but I have learned that there are plenty of things I can do about this." If he begins echoing the feedback he gets at school ("I'm different. I can't do anything right."), get out any supportive evidence you have—his report cards, test scores, artwork, or other concrete forms of achievement—to show him in objective ways how he is making progress.

In some cases, it may also help to focus on your child's effort (how persistent he was or how much thought he gave to the organization) rather than the outcome (what grade he got)— particularly because it is so common for ADHD to involve work production problems. "I'm so proud of you for working so hard on that report" is as powerful a comment, coming from you, as "I'm so proud of you for getting an A." You may also find that it helps to put your child's struggles in context for him. Point out that nearly every child has some type of challenge to overcome—whether it is a learning disability, coordination problems in sports, difficulties with friendships, or a complex home situation.

Reframing negative attitudes goes a long way in helping a child focus on his strengths rather than his disabilities. Your child will also feel much more empowered if you help him develop tools to actively improve the negative situations that disturb him most. Many of the tools for this are similar to those you, your spouse, and your other children have developed yourselves, and sharing your experiences and the responses you have developed will help him feel supported and understood. Your child's pediatrician or counselor can also help him practice specific techniques. For example, many children are advised to deal with teasing by ignoring it, yet ignoring or displaying a sense of anger rarely works, and often even escalates the teasing. Reframing the teasing by turning it into a joke or putting a humorous spin on it can be much more effective. (If teasing becomes a major problem, it needs to be dealt with at school. See Chapter 7.)

Demystifying the nature and treatment of ADHD can be very helpful because children often see their diagnosis as a stigma and their treatment plan as something "done to me" by pediatricians, teachers, and parents instead of seeing themselves as active participants and acknowledging their own successes. Help your child understand that he can shift from perceiving himself as a victim of this disorder to recognizing that he can actually learn to master many areas of difficulty. His pediatrician's explanations about the nature of ADHD— that it has no relation to intelligence, that it is a disorder that can be managed, that many successful adults have this condition—may also help reduce some of his major concerns. At the same time, remind him that other adults in his life—including his teachers and his relatives—are supportive and can serve as advocates for his well-being.

Often the issue of taking medication is especially sensitive. Your child may initially feel devastated by the prospect of taking medication for a "brain problem." He may worry a great deal about other kids' or adults' reactions should they learn he is taking stimulants. He may even assume that this treatment decision means there is "something wrong" with him, that he is "stupid," "weird," or "different" from everyone else. Educating your child about how stimulants work—in any brain, not just in those with ADHD—can demystify some of his fears and help him feel more positive about treatment.

Beyond these steps, you can emphasize to your child that medication is a tool that he can use—like glasses for a person with poor vision who is learning to read, or a hammer for a carpenter building a house. Instead of thinking of himself as a passive recipient being "fixed" or "cured" with stimulants, your child needs to understand the active role he must take in improving his functioning while using medication as a tool that allows him to focus better than before. The more you can encourage him to learn how to use and to take advantage of medication, rather than relying on it to "take care of him," the more progress he is likely to make—and the better he is likely to feel about himself as he learns just how well he can do.

Integrating ADHD Management Into Your Family's Life

Successfully managing ADHD takes a great deal of time and effort on your part as well as your child's. If you, your partner, or any of your other children also have ADHD (not unlikely because the condition can run in families), the amount of time and effort spent is further compounded. Family members without ADHD may resent the time and attention that they feel are taken from them to meet the needs and address the issues of those who have it. It is no surprise, then, that the pressure to satisfy everyone's demands sometimes becomes overwhelming.

One way around this is to formally schedule regular personal time with each child and with your spouse as well. These periods do not have to be lengthy—half an hour at a time may do—but they should be frequent and as predictable (daily, for example) as possible, and you should make sure they actually happen. When you are spending time with one of your children or your spouse, make it a policy not to bring up divisive issues. Try to keep your time positive and focused on the present relationship so that both of you will have more emotional energy for the rest of the family later on. If you are the parent taking most of the responsibility for dealing with issues related to ADHD, it is also a good idea to try to delegate other daily chores as much as possible. Allow your partner, older children, or other relatives to take over duties that free up your time and, when possible, take advantage of time-saving services such as online banking, drive-through services, and so on. Every minute you save from these errands is a valuable minute you can give to your child with ADHD, other family members and, just as important, yourself.

Partnering in Your Child's Care Management

Becoming your child's care manager means serving as the vital link connecting all aspects of his treatment plan at home, at school, and in the community. This requires a great deal of thought, organization, and support, and can make an enormous contribution to your child's progress and your family's welfare. Organization needs to extend beyond some of the aspects already discussed, such as calendars and time management. For example, a child with ADHD accumulates a lot of records—from teachers, physicians, mental health professionals, medical insurance companies, and so on. Keep these papers neatly filed and available when you need them. By organizing reports and treatment decisions chronologically, you can create an excellent database for future discussions with treatment providers and school personnel about how your child is progressing. Always keep a pen and pad of paper or your handheld device available as well to record any information you feel might be useful at the next treatment review meeting with your child's pediatrician. Because concrete, quantitative information is so valuable in evaluating his progress, you will want specific notes on your child's behavior rather than general, half-remembered impressions. Once you have instituted these organizing principles, you will likely find that you have more complete records than any of your child's physicians, psychologists, or teachers, and that you have indeed become the true care manager. Whenever possible, partner with the care manager in your medical home.

In caring for your child with ADHD, the American Academy of Pediatrics recommends creating a "medical home" (see pages 39–40). This term and concept is gaining increasing attention among pediatricians and parents. Despite the name, a medical home is not a building, nor is it a house. Instead, it is an approach to providing your child with high-quality, comprehensive care. It is an ongoing partnership between your family and your pediatrician and other members of your treatment team, and is based on the needs of the whole child and his family. It is defined as care that is coordinated, accessible, continuous, comprehensive, family-centered, compassionate, and culturally effective.

TIPS ON MANAGING HEALTH CARE AND SCHOOL RECORDS

- Create a profile of your child that will follow your child through his years in school as needed.

- Keep a 3-ring binder with dividers. Each divided section can relate to a section on health care, school records, testing, school educational plans, interventions implemented at school (dated and progress noted), and recorded or documented notes with school personnel.

- Keep a 2- to 3-page summary of your child's history, testing, and other findings in the front of this binder. These will often be available from major evaluations that your child has undergone, or as part of his medical home. This will help to ensure that you don't need to reinvent this story for every new provider or treatment resource.

- Keep a summary page for dates of medications used, doses of medications, and positive and negative responses to the medications. This can be invaluable when changes are needed.

- Where possible, find out how to access this information in your child's electronic medical record.

Educating Family Members

While you, your child with ADHD, and other adults involved in his care have probably focused a great deal of attention on learning about the nature of his condition, it is important to keep in mind that your other children and relatives are likely to understand much less. They will need your help in learning how to respond to your child's behavior and to support his efforts to function successfully. If family members seem to resent or blame your child for his actions, take the time to talk privately with them about the challenges he faces. Discuss treatment decisions with everyone in your family, explaining the reasons for your choices. If you are implementing behavior therapy techniques in your home, other family caregivers will need to learn to implement them as well. (Fortunately, all the tools and techniques you will learn through parent training apply equally well to other children in the family and can be equally helpful.) Teach other family members to frame ADHD-related challenges positively and to work with your child to solve problems. You might ask them to write down any issues they have (such as, "Frances interrupts me all the time!") and then think about how to rephrase them in ways that will help solve the problem ("I need for Frances to wait until I'm finished talking before she talks."). Once this is done, family members

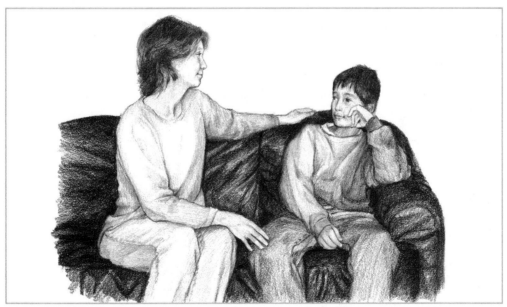

Take time to talk about treatment decisions with everyone in your family so you can help to avoid feelings of resentment and stress.

can discuss possible solutions, try one out and evaluate it, and move on to another solution if that one does not work (see Chapter 6).

Sometimes family members refuse to cooperate, express chronic resentment, or seem unable to act in positive ways. These are common issues; you might consider locating an ADHD support group in your area and/or seeking family therapy to help everyone adjust. In the meantime, let your child communicate directly to his other family members whenever possible instead of always "defending him" yourself. Such conversations can be quite effective in smoothing relationships and helping your child become a respected part of the family.

Taking Care of Yourself

As difficult as it can be at times, it is vital to do whatever you can to avoid letting all the issues you are dealing with interfere significantly with your own sense of competency and well-being. Temporary resentment and stress are inevitable in any challenging family situation, but it is best to just let these moments "roll over" you while doing what you can to address the underlying issues. If you are criticized for poor parenting or your child with ADHD fails to meet his behavior goals, try not to take it personally. Giving both of you credit for trying—and maintaining a sense of humor—can get you through many a difficult day. If you are feeling chronically anxious or depressed, be sure to talk with a psychologist or other mental health counselor. You may benefit from stress management techniques and "reframing" approaches similar to those you used to improve your child's understanding of his ADHD. For example, by reframing "I handled that situation so poorly. It just goes to show what a terrible parent I am" to "I'm glad I reviewed the way I handled that. I can definitely find a better solution" you can transform thoughts that interfere with your functioning to thoughts that facilitate it.

You may also find it stressful at first to carry out some of the behavior management techniques that you will learn in Chapter 6—such as actively ignoring your child's undesirable behavior. Mental and physical relaxation or other techniques can help you learn to remove yourself emotionally in healthy ways during these times. For example, if you are about to react to a situation that you know you should really ignore, you can run through a "mental tape" telling yourself, "OK, stop. Relax. What are my choices? What is my best response?"

Reminding yourself to stop and relax, and to think about whether a particular response is the best way to accomplish your goal, can put some time and space between your impulse to react and your understanding of why you should ignore that particular behavior. This type of technique allows you to make better choices and set an example of sound behavior management for your child.

If you find that the stress of parenting a child with ADHD has caused problems in your relationship with your spouse or partner, do not hesitate to seek marital or couples counseling to address any ongoing problems. Keep in mind that ignoring problematic issues rarely makes them go away. Your, and your partner's, physical and emotional health must remain top priority—not only for your child's sake, but also for your own.

Peer Relationships: Getting Along With Other Children

It can be painful to observe the insensitive ways in which children with ADHD are sometimes treated by their peers. Your child may long to be one of the "popular" kids and, while this may not always be a fully realistic option, you can do a lot to help him make friends and work cooperatively with others. Social relationships are critical to address and important to long-term adjustment, but difficult to change. Social skills counseling or formal group instruction can often be ineffective because children with ADHD can find it difficult to transfer a skill that they have learned in therapy or in a class to their everyday school environment, unless they are given all the tools and ample opportunity to practice how to use them. Social skills programs offered at schools or in settings like intensive summer camp programs may be more effective because the child interacts in class with other children in the actual setting similar to those he encounters every day. The training is most successful if it allows the child to practice new skills first in the social skills class and then prompts him to use them in supervised natural settings, such as the playground—and also provides rewards for their appropriate use. Programs such as special therapeutic summer camps (see Chapter 7) for children with ADHD are particularly effective for teaching social skills and sports competencies that can improve peer relationships. You can also provide structure or "scaffolding" for a young child by scheduling play dates with his peers, allowing him to develop social skills in a comfortable setting. At first keep the play dates short and have a parent-supervised agenda, such as first baking cookies together and then playing a board game that you already know is handled well by your child. As time passes and he becomes more successful in relating to peers, you can gradually remove that scaffolding and let him enjoy growing relationships with less of your own involvement. After these kinds of play dates you may want to sit down with your child and debrief: "I liked it a lot when you decided to let David choose the game. I could see that it made him really happy," or "When Jessica started grabbing the Barbies for herself, what do you think are some of the things that you could have done?"

As social skills improve, your guidance within the context of your child's daily life will continue to be an important tool in helping him improve social relationships. Many of the techniques that parents use with any child can be used in a more focused, deliberate way to help your child with ADHD. While all parents teach acceptable social behavior by modeling it themselves, you may want to be especially sure you are demonstrating certain skills, including using appropriate body language that you hope your child will learn every time you interact with him. Narrating your behavior as you interact with your child can also set a good example ("Here, Joanie, I'll let you have a turn now. We get along better when we take turns.") and help your child focus on the issue at hand. Meanwhile, keep an eye out for—and strictly limit or eliminate—such negative social interactions as seen on violent television shows or computer or video games, violent and inappropriate behavior in other family members, and overaggressive playmates.

Older children can benefit from conversations about particular issues and from your interpreting social interactions as they happen ("It makes me angry when you take food from my plate without asking. I feel like you don't respect my rights as a person. Now I'm going to ask you to put it back."). Many parents also find it helpful to reward their child's progress in targeted social interactions with stickers or other small rewards. Small fines or loss of privileges for violating important social rules may prove effective too.

Finally, one of the best ways to boost your child's self-esteem is to encourage him to participate in extracurricular social activities that are set up to foster positive peer relationships (such as Scouts, sports teams, and church youth groups). The key to your child's success in these extracurricular activities is to have them supervised by adults who are familiar with ADHD and know how to apply the principles of behavior therapy (see Chapter 6). Parents can be better and more effective soccer coaches for your child and all team members if they use effective behavior management techniques. Becoming part of a small group or team under these conditions can be a great morale booster as your child experiments with making friends in a safe, supervised setting. Such groups can be especially effective if they involve an activity your child especially enjoys or is good at because he can then rely on his skill to help make up for any social weaknesses. Again, summer programs that focus on peer relationships and on sports skills can be particularly helpful in this regard. If your child is taking stimulant medication, he may find that the medication helps him considerably in controlling his impulsivity in these types of social situations and allows him to participate more fully. If his daily long-acting medication has worn off by the time his group activity begins, the option of an extra short-term dose half an hour before the meeting begins may help him participate more fully.

Seeking Out Other Positive Relationships

Many children with ADHD have difficulty making friends among children their age. If you sense that your child feels lonely and isolated, even after trying some of the social skills techniques outlined previously, consider also the people in your community who might serve as positive role models, supportive mentors, or friends. An older teenager or adult who shares one or more of your child's interests and understands how his overactivity or impulsivity interfere with his social relationships can make a huge difference in his self-esteem by just listening carefully and offering empathy and advice. Even if your child has a positive, supportive relationship with you, having another adult or older teenager in more of a mentor role can be quite beneficial, because this is a different kind of relationship with a unique payoff. Search among your relatives and friends for a responsible person who might be willing to provide this support for your child. If none is available, ask your local ADHD support group for leads or advice. Your religious institution, local social service agency, or mentoring organization (such as Big Brothers/Big Sisters) may be another source of help.

Finally, keep in mind that your own presence means a great deal to your child—not just when engaged in practical activities but when both of you are free to just play or hang out together. Your supportive presence, sharing an activity, or just talking lets your child know that you love and like to be with him and can help to balance social disappointment that he may have experienced elsewhere. Sometimes children with ADHD view their parents as the only people consistently in their corner. In addition to providing your child with social and emotional benefits, a close, positive relationship can make you a more effective reinforcer, leading to a decrease in disciplinary problems.

Being Your Child's Best Advocate

As you discover new ways to facilitate positive behaviors, learning, and self-esteem in your child, be sure to pass these techniques on to the other people in his life—adults in your household, other caregivers, relatives, teachers and, when appropriate, even empathetic peers or siblings—so that they can help maintain the consistency, structure, and clarity your child needs. If necessary, remind them that ADHD is a neurobehavioral disorder, not the result of poor discipline, and that specific, consistent, positive techniques and attitudes can help to improve a child's ability to manage his own behavior. Show caregivers and close relatives how to implement the techniques you have learned and talk with them periodically about how your child is responding and what, if any, changes they have observed. Remember, all of these adults in your child's life should be thought of as part of the team that helps him adjust to and manage the ADHD behaviors and challenges. If they become partners, your child will progress more rapidly than if you were in conflict with teachers, caregivers, and others at every turn. You can read a great deal more about advocacy in Chapter 8.

A PARENT'S STORY

A Support System

"One of the worst aspects of having ADHD for my daughter was the fact that it seemed like no one else in our area had it," writes one mother. "The other kids at school called her 'crazy' all the time, and I think she really believed she would never be OK. Then, when she was about nine, we got her a computer and linked her up to a couple of ADHD Web sites. She started reading some of the bulletin boards and 'personal stories' and also using some of the 'ask the experts' options. We made sure that the sites she visited were responsible. After a while we saw her attitude really start to change. Not only had she learned a lot of really valuable information about ADHD on the Internet, she also began to feel less isolated and more supported. I don't know how she would have gotten through junior high and high school without that computer. Those resources gave her the confidence she needed to get through school."

Mary, Wooster, OH

The symptoms of ADHD can seem so overwhelming at first that many parents fear there is nothing they can do to provide substantial help for their child. Yet while it is true that treating ADHD and managing its symptoms requires time, patience, and a great deal of attention, the benefits can be enormous to family functioning and family relations. Attending treatment review meetings with your child's pediatrician, implementing behavior therapy techniques, talking with your child about the challenges he experiences, and providing him with resources may seem like tiny steps on the road to better functioning, but together they really do have a positive impact. Children, who naturally want most of all to be like every other child, often tend to resist thinking about or wanting to address the issues that ADHD symptoms impose. Therefore, it is up to you to provide your child with the services he needs, the extras that can so greatly improve his daily life, and the support and education he needs to see them as useful tools for him.

For your entire family's sake as well as your child's, stay up to date on the latest research on ADHD, engage your child's teachers in his evaluation and treatment plan, and do what you can to help your child learn to recognize his own strengths and manage his own targeted problems. With the help and guidance of physicians, a therapist, counselors, teachers, and other professional advisors, you can make an enormous difference in your child's life. Adults with ADHD successfully attend college, marry, have families, and enjoy fulfilling careers—thanks in large part to the parents who took the time and made the effort to help them navigate their journey.

Q & A

Q: *My nine-year-old son was recently diagnosed with ADHD. He seems to be responding well to treatment and discussions of what ADHD is and how he can work to manage his problems. However, his older sister, who is thirteen, has responded to the news much more negatively. She resists going anywhere with the family where she might be seen by classmates in the company of her brother. At home, she calls him "weird" and yells at him to stay away from her and her friends. I understand that it can be difficult for an adolescent to deal with anything "different" about her family, but her behavior is rude and is damaging to my son's self-esteem, hard as we are working to build it up. What can we do to persuade our daughter to be more supportive of her brother?*

A: It may help to look at a situation like this as more of an opportunity than a problem because it gives you an opening to work with your daughter on general issues relating to sensitivity to others, respect for family members' rights and feelings, and acceptance of the challenges that each person must face, as well as issues directly related to ADHD. As you are already doing with your son, your daughter needs to be educated regarding what ADHD is and is not, which of your son's behaviors are typical of children with ADHD and which are just part of normal sibling conflicts, and how her responses can help him achieve better self-control and improve general family functioning. If you have not already spoken directly with your daughter about these issues, be sure to do so—you might do some of this in the context of a "family meeting." Your family may also benefit from one or more sessions with a family therapist or from a support group for families of children with ADHD that may help your daughter understand that the problems that she faces with her brother are common, and provide her with positive approaches for interacting with her brother.

Q: *Our eleven-year-old daughter, who has been diagnosed with inattentive-type ADHD, has been doing better since she began treatment with stimulant medication. However, we still have trouble getting her organized around homework. We have tried setting up an office in her room, taking away all the distractions, keeping the area quiet, and not allowing the television to go on until all her homework is done. We don't seem to be making much progress and, in fact, we are all getting even more frustrated because nothing seems to work. Her teachers still complain that work is not getting turned in, and her grades are still suffering in spite of her teacher always telling us how bright she is.*

A: There is no one-size-fits-all solution to the ideal homework setting. Some children with ADHD work inefficiently in an isolated, quiet setting like their room, and do better in the midst of some action, like at the kitchen table with a radio playing. You might need to try a few different settings until you find the most efficient one. In addition, you might need to figure out if any other factors are making homework difficult. Think about all the steps involved. Does your child know what all the assignments are? Does she bring the materials home that are necessary for doing the work? Does she have a nightly work plan that fits with her learning style? (She might need to schedule breaks between math and English, or between outlining the report and writing the first 3 paragraphs.) Does she have a system to check on whether all the nightly work is done? Is there a system for checking that her completed work gets turned in on the due date? How does she or you know that work is late? Have you or her teacher set up rewards for progress or consequences for late work? Is there a system for her teacher to communicate with you about late work? Once you have gone through this type of systematic list of questions, you can begin to solve the problem in an organized way—and you might discover some simple and obvious solutions. If she is taking stimulant medication and she does her homework primarily at a time after it has worn off, you could consider a short-acting extended dose of medication for the early evening.

Chapter 6

Behavior Therapy: Parenting Techniques That Work

Many parents discover that their child with attention-deficit/hyperactivity disorder (ADHD) does not respond to parenting efforts that they used successfully with their other children. The failure to comply with family rules or expectations can be especially upsetting because it leads others to assume that a child's behavior is due to faulty parenting rather than a diagnosed condition. Your negative experiences with your child may convince you that she is unable to understand or to remember your instructions and therefore can never improve her behavior.

In fact, your child with ADHD is likely as able to comprehend and retain what you tell her as her siblings are. But because she has difficulties with the ability to control her actions, organize her thoughts, think before she acts, or create a plan of action and follow through, she may not be able to *perform* in a way she knows is appropriate. She may understand, for example, that it is not right to interrupt you repeatedly while you are talking on the phone, or to wander away when you are talking to her, but be unable to stop herself. The way she operates may seem more like, "ready…fire…aim!"—she thinks about the rules after she has already broken them instead of before. This is why some of the parenting approaches that worked with your other children may be ineffective. Again, it is not that your child does not know what the appropriate behaviors are, it is just hard for her to carry them out.

At present, behavior therapy, a form of therapy taught to parents as *behavioral parent training,* has been proven to be reliably effective in moving children with ADHD from understanding appropriate behavior to actually functioning in more positive ways. This form of therapy focuses on (1) helping parents acquire parenting skills and behaviors and (2) decreasing children's aggressive, noncompliant, or hyperactive behaviors. The Centers for Disease Control and Prevention has recently reviewed parent training techniques that lead to better outcome for families and children, as well as components of programs that are less effective.

Successful methods of helping parents acquire parenting skills and behaviors and emotional communication skills include

- Teaching parents active listening skills, such as reflecting back what the child is saying This also teaches parents to help children recognize their feelings, label their emotions, and appropriately express and deal with emotions. This may also involve teaching parents to reduce negative communication patterns (sarcasm and criticism) and allowing children to feel like they are equal contributors to the communication process.
- Teaching parents to interact positively with their child
- Requiring parents to practice with their child during program sessions

Successful methods of decreasing children's aggressive, noncompliant, or hyperactive behaviors include

- Teaching parents to interact positively with their child and decrease unwanted behaviors by praising positives and ignoring most negatives
- Teaching parents the correct use of time-out
- Teaching parents to respond consistently to their child
- Requiring parents to practice with their child during program sessions

Less effective components of parent training programs include

- Teaching parents how to problem-solve about child behaviors
- Teaching parents how to promote children's academic and cognitive skills
- Including ancillary services as part of the parenting program

---

A PARENT'S STORY

Parenting Approaches

"It was difficult to understand at first why my parenting approach had so little effect with my youngest, Suzanne, who has ADHD," a mother writes. "I treated her the same way I treated all my other kids, but it seemed like every time I figured out how to help her change her behavior in a positive direction she'd fall back into her old habits before the week was up. She was also a lot angrier and more defiant than her older sisters. By the time she was diagnosed with ADHD, I was
at my wits' end. Nothing I tried with her—talking, rewarding, punishing—seemed to work. It was only after I went through the parent training instruction recommended by her pediatrician that I started to understand why many of my approaches were not effective and how I could work systematically to shape her behavior."

Gail, Milwaukee, WI

Parent training's emphasis on ways in which adults can better understand, manage, and shape their child's behavior differs from other approaches that focus directly on the child and are designed to change her emotional status (such as traditional psychotherapy) or patterns of thinking (such as cognitive-behavioral therapy). These latter approaches have not been found consistently helpful in the treatment of ADHD. In this chapter, you will be introduced to the principles underlying behavior therapy for families of children with ADHD. You will learn

- What behavior therapy consists of, who it is for, and where it is available
- Which specific parenting techniques have been found to be effective in improving children's functioning and how they must be implemented
- How the gains achieved through behavior therapy techniques can be preserved

Behavior therapy techniques are often taught in highly structured 7- to 12-week individual or group parent training sessions by therapists or specially trained and certified instructors, usually consisting of one session per week. Such courses have been shown to be effective for families with ADHD because they allow for weekly feedback—letting parents ask questions and receive helpful advice from the instructor—and may offer parents the chance to share their experiences with others in similar situations. Unfortunately, while parent training is now available in many communities, it may not be in yours, or may be available but not be covered by your insurance plan. Even if this is the case, by reading the material in this chapter you should be able to apply many of these principles in your daily interactions with your child. But you may find it even more useful to work with a child therapist or your child's pediatrician to adapt these techniques to your own unique situation even if it is not in the exact systematic approach described here.

What Is Behavior Therapy, Who Is It For, and Where Is It Available?

Simply put, behavior therapy/behavioral parent training consists of a set of practical, tested procedures designed to provide you with the strategies you need to improve family interactions and your child's ability to manage his behavior. Parent training is just that—a program aimed at training you, the parents, to successfully manage and shape your child's behavior. By focusing less on the child's emotional state and more on his actual behaviors, it attempts to turn parents into their child's "therapist" by teaching them how to encourage and maintain positive behaviors, determine which behaviors can be actively ignored, and know when and how to set and enforce rules. All forms of behavior therapy, including parent training, share a common set of principles and offer an array of techniques that can be combined in different ways to help increase a child's abilities for self-regulation. A sound parent training program should help you

- Gain a better understanding of what behaviors are normal for your child.
- Learn to achieve consistent and positive interactions.
- Cut down on negative interactions, such as arguing or constantly having to repeat instructions.
- Provide appropriate consequences for your child's behavior.
- Become more empathetic of your child's viewpoint.
- Assist your child in improving her abilities to manage her own behaviors.

Who Benefits Most From Behavior Therapy?

In most cases, the younger your child is, the more successful a behavior therapy program is likely to be because it is easier to change negative behaviors that have not been in place for very long. (Still, even teenagers can benefit from a sound and consistent behavioral approach. See Chapter 11.) Because behavioral parent training requires sufficient verbal skills for your child to understand what you are telling her, and to discuss her present behavior patterns and the plan for behavior change, it usually is recommended for families when the child is at least preschool-aged. Children who have more serious conduct problems may need additional professional help, or a different type of help, to improve their functioning.

Behavior therapy may be most effective in some situations when it is used along with stimulant medication that allows the child to be more fully attentive to the techniques being introduced. Combining medication management with behavior therapy can, in many cases, modestly but significantly increase the chances that parents and teachers will regard a child's behavior as comparable to that of children who do not have ADHD. For children who have ADHD without coexisting conditions (Chapter 9) and have adequate social functioning, and few significant behavioral problems, well-planned and monitored medication management may be the best treatment option. For preschoolers, children, and youth who have ADHD complicated by oppositional symptoms, poor social functioning, and behavior problems from suboptimal or negative parenting practices, a combination of medication management and behavior therapy has been found to be the most effective treatment option. For toddlers and preschoolers with oppositional and behaviors with or without ADHD, behavioral parent training/behavioral therapy is the suggested first line of treatment.

Whether or not your child is taking medication, behavior therapy may help improve your relationship with her. Parents and children report greater satisfaction when behavior therapy is included in their overall treatment plan, and in some cases the benefits of parent training include being able to reduce the dose of stimulant medication needed to achieve targeted behavioral goals. An additional benefit of parent training is that the principles work well for all children in the family, not just for children with ADHD, and adopting a parenting approach that uses these techniques can lead to better overall family relationships.

Coexisting Conditions and Family Issues

If your child has been diagnosed with ADHD and other coexisting conditions, her pediatrician can help you determine the behavioral treatment priorities for your child based on her individual needs. For example, if your child has been diagnosed with ADHD and also has anxiety, either behavior therapy or medication management may lead to similar gains. However, children with ADHD and oppositional and defiant or conduct disorder may benefit more from treatment that combines both medication and behavior therapy rather than medication alone. Although intensive behavioral therapy is the first-line and most effective treatment for children with autism spectrum disorders, children who have ADHD symptoms in addition may need a different approach to medication management for these symptoms than children who have ADHD alone. Children with ADHD and severe depression may also require different medication management and a different type of behavioral treatment plan. The kind of parent training described in this chapter may also not be appropriate in these situations.

Ideally, at the time that your child was diagnosed with ADHD, any coexisting disorders were also identified. Keep in mind, though, that certain conditions may escape notice early on or only surface at a later time. If your child exhibits symptoms that make you suspect she has a disruptive behavior disorder, depression, or anxiety, discuss your concerns with her pediatrician. It may be necessary to reconsider her diagnosis and coexisting conditions and to change her treatment plan accordingly.

Family circumstances may also affect your ability to make gains using behavior therapy techniques. If communication among members of your family is extremely difficult; you are experiencing serious marital problems; or family members are struggling with multiple major issues, including any form of family violence, parent training may not work for you. In these circumstances, meeting with a psychotherapist for family therapy may be a more helpful strategy.

Where Can I Find a Parent Training Program?

If behavioral parent training programs exist in your community and are covered by your health insurance, your child's pediatrician can point you toward an appropriate resource. Check to be sure that the therapist or training leader is a qualified mental health or other medical professional and that the program follows a systematic format adapted specifically for parents of children with ADHD. It can be useful to check to see if a particular behavior therapist is certified by the American Board of Psychology. Your own pediatrician or mental health resource, or developmental and behavioral or mental health departments at your local children's hospital, may be able to help you find some resources. The best programs are evidence-based—they have already been found effective through carefully conducted research. While less standardized parent training programs may be available, they are not as likely to be as helpful for families dealing with ADHD.

Some schools have been able to fund and train their teachers in the use of behavior therapy techniques. If your child's teacher is able to participate in such courses, she and your child would probably benefit enormously. By participating in parent training with your partner and sharing behavior therapy strategies with your child's other caregivers (including her teacher), you can help others support your child's efforts to meet the target outcomes that you and the rest of her treatment team have identified.

If no formal parent training programs are presently available in your community, you can still apply these principles to the specifics of your own situation, and may be able to use this information to advocate for the development of these services through your child's pediatrician, your school system, or other local agencies or support groups. Take the time to review the information that follows in this chapter, and think about the ways in which you may be able to incorporate these practices into your daily life with your child.

Behavior Therapy: The Specifics of Parent Training

Research confirms that behavioral parent training programs are valuable tools to help parents guide, support, and live more comfortably with their children with ADHD. Behavior therapy is different from psychological interventions directed to the child and designed to change the child's emotional status (eg, play therapy) or thought patterns (eg, cognitive therapy or cognitive-behavioral therapy). These psychological interventions do not have a demonstrated effect on the outcome of children with ADHD, and gains achieved in the treatment setting usually do not transfer into the classroom or home. By contrast, behavioral parent training and similar classroom behavior interventions have successfully changed the behavior of children with ADHD. These programs are considered by researchers and the American Academy of Pediatrics (AAP) to be first-line proven treatment approaches for children with ADHD. Following are brief descriptions of some topics and techniques that parent training programs introduce through direct instruction, demonstrations, role-playing, readings, discussions, and "homework assignments" that parents can use with their own child.

Learning the Basics

As you begin a parent training program it is important to ground yourself in basic information about ADHD and the causes of oppositional and defiant behavior. As well as reading books such as this and visiting responsible Web sites, your therapist or coach should include information about these topics as you embark on behavioral parent training instruction.

Setting the Stage for Behavior Change: Learning How to Spend Positive Time or "Hang Out" With Your Child

Behavior therapy is not just about a child's behavior, but about improving the relationships between a child and her parents (as well as others) and the interactions within the family. As a parent, you can take the first step toward improved relationships by understanding how discouraging your child's daily experiences can be to her and by countering that negativity with positive messages and support.

Many parent training programs suggest that establishing a positive playtime is a very helpful first step in setting the stage for successful outcomes. You can do this by setting aside a short period each day to play with your child, during which you refrain from giving instructions or commands or asking questions and, alternatively, imitate what your child is doing, describing what she is doing, with enthusiasm. During this time, your goal is not to teach your child anything or to shape her behavior. It is to let her know that you are interested in her and want to spend time getting to know her better. This can be accomplished by announcing that from now on you will reserve time during several days each week to be with your child (her other parent should do the same) and, during this time, allow her to decide on the activity (any activity that allows the 2 of you to interact is fine—such as playing with board games or dolls, but not watching television or playing organized sports). While you are involved in the activity, allow your child to take the lead. Comment occasionally to show you are paying attention and are involved, and provide positive feedback now and then, but do not try to take over the activity or conversation. The point is to simply be with your child—to let her be the center of your attention and to show you her world. By regularly participating in these activities with your child you are learning to listen and observe while avoiding constantly giving commands or instructions—the first skills necessary to begin reshaping her behavior and changing her relationships within the family. You are also demonstrating in the most effective way possible that your child does not need to engage in negative behaviors to win your attention. Once she learns she has her parents' interest, she can rely on this in trusting them to help her figure out how to get along better and develop more positive relationships with others.

Responding Effectively to Your Child's Behavior

Once you and your child have begun to establish a basis of trust and positive support, it is time to look at the ways you hope to improve your interactions with her at home. Parent interactions can be improved, and improved interactions can set the stage for the successful use of parent training tools and techniques. One of the first principles of parent training is to expand the notion of the word *discipline.* Many parents assume that the term refers to ways to carry out effective punishment. However, teaching discipline to a child really means teaching self-control—and that is the broad goal of parent training. Fortunately, behavior therapy programs take a more positive approach than just constantly devising punishments for breaking rules. As your child's "teacher-coach-therapist," you will learn how to choose the most effective response to any given situation.

In most cases, you will find that you have 3 choices when confronted with a particular behavior in your child: you can *praise* the behavior, deliberately *ignore* it, or *punish* your child for it. Behavioral parent training will help you to decide which response to choose, how to follow up on that decision, and how to become consistent about your choices from one event, and one day, to the next. Of course, it is not always easy to decide whether a behavior deserves to be ignored or punished, and it is not always obvious when and how to provide praise. These and other topics will be discussed in this chapter. In the meantime, though, it is important to consider how much more powerful and, in most cases, preferable positive reinforcement and ignoring are to punishment, even though in the heat of the moment this may go against your instincts or intuition. It may help to think about how much more likely you are to work hard when your supervisor at work recognizes and praises your efforts, and how poorly motivated and resentful you may feel if she frequently criticizes you. In the same way, your child is more likely to respond positively to your actions if you react positively to her, while a negative comment or response on your part is likely to lead to more negative behavior. This is why in behavioral parent training, parents are encouraged to praise their child's behavior whenever possible, and ignore it when necessary, as a strong way of shaping behavior while minimizing the need for punishment.

THREE BASIC RULES

When Responding to Your Child's Behavior

Many parents making use of behavior therapy techniques find it helpful to rely on the following simple rules when interacting with their child:

- If you want to see a behavior continue, praise it.
- If you do not like a behavior but it is not dangerous or intolerable, ignore it.
- If you have to stop a behavior that is dangerous or intolerable (for instance, your child hitting a sibling to hurt her, not just to get your attention), punish it.

Giving Clear Commands

The first step in helping your child learn to follow rules, obey your commands, and otherwise manage her own behavior is to make sure that the commands you give her are clear. Adults are often accustomed to couching their commands in a variety of "softening" or ambiguous gestures and phrases. Many of us also tend to react too strongly or impulsively to behavior we consider unacceptable. But children with ADHD need to be told what to do in a clear, straightforward, and nonemotional way if they are to learn to control their actions. You can give effective commands by

- **Establishing good eye contact.** You must fully engage your child's attention by making good eye contact if she is going to hear and follow what you say. At first, you may find it helpful to touch a younger child's arm or hold her hand before addressing her.
- **Clearly stating the command.** You can make commands clear to your child by first stating what behavior therapists call a *terminating command*—a simple, nonemotional statement of what you want your child to do ("You need to stop pushing your brother."). If the behavior does not stop immediately, you can then follow up with a *warning* that includes the exact limit and the *consequences* ("If you push your brother one more time, you'll be in time-out. If you stop immediately, the two of you can go on playing."). When stating a command, keep your tone of voice firm and neutral. Refrain from yelling, or looking or sounding angry. It is especially important to monitor your body language because these nonverbal messages are so easy for parents to overlook. State the command

as an instruction, not as a question (Not, "Would you please stop teasing your brother?" or "Stop teasing him, OK?" but "You need to stop teasing your brother.").

If you are not sure your child heard the terminating command or warning, ask her to repeat it back to you. Then pay attention to whether she carries out your instructions and respond immediately to her behavior. If she responds as you have asked, respond positively with praise, thanks, a thumbs-up, a high five, or other acknowledgment that she has done well. If her response is not exactly what you had hoped for but is in the right direction, offer her immediate praise for the part of your command that she did carry out. If your child does not start to respond according to the limits you have set ("one more time" or "within the next two minutes") invoke the consequences that you have already set, calmly narrating what is happening as you do so ("You did not stop pushing your brother, so you'll have the five-minute time-out that we just talked about.") Keep in mind that because you have given a warning and a terminating command and spelled out the consequences for complying or disobeying, if she does not follow your instructions you have not "put her in" the time-out—*she* has "chosen" the time-out for herself as an alternative to following your command. This is a key point. If you give your child a command, she doesn't comply, and you immediately "put her" in time-out, you have skipped the step of her choosing whether to receive the positive or negative consequence. You have lost an opportunity to teach her self-control. Remember the bottom line of whether a parenting principle is sound: DOES IT TEACH SELF-CONTROL?

If you make a point of following through on the positive or negative consequences of each command, every time, you should soon find that you will not have to repeat your instructions over and over as you probably did before. Your ultimate goal will be to give a command only once for it to be obeyed. Parents are often concerned that "I have to say it eight times before she does it." Children are thinking, "the first seven times are free! Then she gets angry and I finally have to do it." The elimination of constant pleading, nagging, or threatening is a great relief to most parents and goes a long way toward improving their interaction with their child. If you are tempted to "let it slide" when she ignores a command (telling yourself, perhaps, that she does have ADHD, after all), consider how hard it will be to make up for this inconsistency in the future and carry out the promised consequences. If you are going to try to follow up on each command you give, you will need to consider beforehand how important the command you are about to give is. Limiting the number of commands you give will make it easier for you to follow up on each and every one, thus increasing your chances of success.

At first, as you practice giving commands according to these guidelines, you will need to keep things simple. Make sure that all your commands are achievable by your child, and wait until she has completed one step of your instructions before giving another. If necessary, break a complex command down into smaller steps ("Take off your shoes. Good job! Now take off your socks."). This can result in your child being able to successfully carry out the command and build on successes, rather than to fail because the command was too complicated and feel like she can "never" do what you ask. While your child is carrying out your instructions, avoid distracting her. Be sure to follow up on each command, avoid giving commands unless you mean for her to follow them (do not tell her to go to bed until it is really time), and stick to commands that you know can be carried out successfully by your child. It is usually best to give a time limit ("by the third time," "by three minutes") for each command as well, to help her focus on accomplishing it and to help you both define when it has or has not been accomplished. Keep in mind, however, that children with ADHD often have particular problems with time awareness and time limits. You will need to keep such limits simple, and consider using egg timers or other creative clock devices to make these time limits more concrete. By doing so, you can turn commands that have previously ended in failure and frustration ("Go upstairs and clean your room.") to commands that end in success and build on your child's self-esteem ("Put your video game player away by the time this bell goes off in three minutes.").

Shaping Behaviors Gradually: Small Steps in the Right Direction Add Up

Children with ADHD, like all of us, will probably have particular difficulty changing a complex or long-standing set of behaviors. Expecting your child to make a major behavioral change all at once will most likely result in frustration and failure for you both. As mentioned previously, you can support your child's efforts to change a complex set of behaviors by breaking the plan down into smaller, achievable steps, and tackling one at a time. This is called "shaping" your child's behavior. The idea is to break down tasks to the point at which each step is achievable and ends in success and praise for your child instead of failure and frustration. Behavioral parent training will help you learn to do this by having you review your targeted outcomes (specific goals) for your child's behavior and ways you can help her achieve them. You as a parent (or other primary caregiver) can start by writing down what you see as each step toward completing a task or correcting a complex behavior and follow up by creating a plan for working on each step, one at a time. You can incorporate your child in the development of each plan at the level that she can appropriately participate. Even minor goals can be broken down in this way. In writing down the steps involved in completing a chore, for example, you might list the steps that your child needs to take in cleaning up his room, such as

- Puts dirty clothes in a hamper
- Puts books away
- Puts toys in the drawers under his bed
- Pulls up the covers

Then you can start with a single command—"You need to start cleaning up your room by putting the dirty clothes in the hamper." When this is done successfully, you can praise her—"Good job!" If you had just said, "You need to clean your room" and she *had* put her clothes in the hamper, but not put her books and toys away and pulled up the covers, she would not have been successful and you would have ended up making a negative remark or giving a consequence. At the point that putting her clothes in the hamper when you ask becomes automatic then, after a few days, you can add the next step—putting the clothes in the hamper and putting her books away, and praising her for the successful completion.

When this is successful you can add the next task, and so on, until the list is complete. In this way you can "shape her behavior" and at the same time turn what used to be negative interactions into positive ones that build on his self-esteem and competence.

You can help your child learn to focus better and accomplish tasks more quickly by timing certain tasks as well and encouraging her to try to break her own speed record again and again. Such small triumphs can mean a great deal to children who have experienced repeated failure or frustration at home or at school. Behavior shaping techniques also heighten your child's awareness of each successful step, helping her to "own" her behavioral successes.

Choosing What to Praise, Ignore, or Punish

The next step in parent training is learning to recognize behaviors that require positive, ignoring, or punishment responses. You will be encouraged to do your best to "catch your child being good" and praise her for it whenever possible because this allows for positive interaction and enhances her relationship with you as it strengthens her positive behaviors. Praise should be simple and straightforward ("I like the way you did that.") and not spoiled

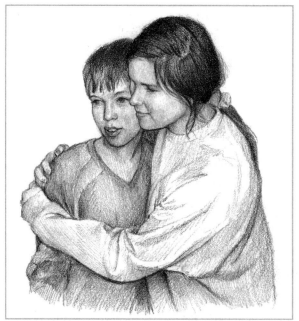

by negative references ("Great job—why can't you always do it like that?")—this is called praise spoiling. In many cases a simple smile, hug, or arm around your child's shoulders is even more effective than words. Such immediate positive reinforcement is actually a much stronger (and less risky) way to change behavior than larger, long-term rewards, such as the offer of a video game system for maintaining all Bs or staying on the honor roll all semester. However,

In many cases a simple smile, hug, or an arm around your child's shoulders is even more effective than words.

you may still decide to offer your child stickers, points in a token reward system, or other prizes for putting in the effort to help change behaviors you are working on as long as you know that your child will be successful at achieving these rewards.

"Active ignoring" is one of the most powerful behavioral tools available to parents, but one of the hardest to carry out. Once you give a command, you must follow it through to the end if it is going to be effective and meaningful to your child. Many parents are in the habit of giving frequent corrections all through the day, and then either do not follow through on many of them or dole out so many punishments that they become ineffective and set up a negative relationship with their child. Learning how to actively ignore certain situations can lead to many fewer commands and significantly improve this situation.

In fact, you may be surprised at how effective ignoring a negative behavior can be. This is especially true once your child has grown accustomed to the positive attention she enjoys in your special times together and no longer needs to demand your attention in negative ways. A child who interrupts your phone conversations over and over is, in most cases, only doing it to get your attention. If you respond by saying something like, "Sarah, I'm on the phone— wait until I get off!" you may think you are giving a command to stop the behavior but you are actually rewarding her by giving her the attention she wanted in the first place. If, instead, you ignore her behavior (by not looking at her or responding in words), her attempts to distract you while you are on the phone may escalate at first, while she tries even harder to get the attention that she is used to. This is what behavior therapists call an "extinction burst"—the behavior gets worse before it gets better. However, if you consistently ignore her, she will gradually learn more functional ways to have her needs met. In this way, ignoring works as a powerful tool for behavior change. A large proportion of behavior problems can be addressed with a combination of praising and ignoring techniques.

As part of a typical parent training program, you will identify the few behaviors that you consider so dangerous (running into the street without looking, for example) or intolerable (hitting other children to hurt them) that they must be met with immediate action or punishment on your part. Your therapist will teach you how to discuss these behaviors with your child ahead of time, figure out the punishments that will follow, and determine possible ways to avoid the same situation in the future. He will help you understand how much more effective punishment can be if it is limited to only your child's most dangerous or intolerable behaviors. When punishment occurs too frequently (as it often does for children with ADHD), its effects are diminished and the child may no longer consistently respond to it. Children can become quite resentful, angry, and negative. Because of this, negative consequences should be reserved for those few instances when parents feel they must do something immediately (and not just ignore). Any punishment should be preceded, whenever possible, by a terminating and a warning signal. That way your child will always have the opportunity to exert self-control and avoid the punishment.

No matter what your response to your child's behavior, it will be most effective if it takes place immediately. Putting off a discussion until later, or offering a reward at the end of the week for general good behavior, will greatly diminish its effect. The response you have chosen to a particular behavior should be as consistent as possible as well. If you responded appropriately to your child's pushing her brother down with punishment yesterday, respond in the same way today. Your parent training therapist will help you decide in advance on the best responses to your child's most frequent behavior issues so you can use these techniques with confidence.

Using Rewards to Motivate Positive Behavior

Praise is a powerful motivator for all children, but many also especially enjoy and respond well to additional, tangible motivators such as reward charts and token economies. Reward charts (contingency charts) usually consist of daily calendar sheets listing 4 or 5 achievable chores, behaviors, or other goals on which you and your child have agreed. Before instituting the reward chart with your child, you will have observed her enough to know that she can successfully complete most of the behaviors listed. The description of each behavior needs to be clear, countable, and unambiguous (for example, "is upstairs brushing his teeth within 5 minutes after being told" or "gets out of bed by the third time she's asked"). You might have 5 items on a chart—4 of which are easily achievable by your child with an additional one that you are presently working on. Charts can be reviewed daily, and this becomes a time to let your child know how proud you are of her for working on her chores or behavior. If too many of the items are not achievable and do not end up with stars or stickers, your child will get easily frustrated and negative about participating. Each time your child accomplishes the goal she receives a sticker, a star, or other mark of achievement on the chart. Many younger children are happy enough just to receive the stickers or stars themselves, but some older children may want to accumulate numbers of stars or stickers and redeem them for privileges—such as a trip to a baseball game or to the beach, or modest, prearranged material rewards. These rewards do not need to be new privileges. What you are really doing is putting some of her everyday privileges under her behavioral control, knowing in advance that she will experience success. The table on page 126 summarizes some of the key concepts described in this section.

Another type of reward system, called a token economy, also involves receiving tokens, stars, stickers, or points for behaving appropriately or complying with commands. Token economies are similar to reward charts in that they can often be helpful when praise alone is not enough to motivate a child to complete tasks or stick to routines. The gains from using a token economy approach can often be seen quickly, but can also fade unless this kind of system is kept up for some time. Each targeted behavior is given a value (3 stickers, 4 points) depending on how difficult a challenge it is for your child. You and your child can then create a list of fun activities or treats that she can "buy" with a prearranged number of stickers or points. Response cost—the withdrawing of rewards or privileges in response to unwanted or problem behavior—can be eventually added onto this system if necessary. In that case, your child's failure to accomplish a targeted behavior on her own or after an agreed-on limit results in the same number of stickers or points being deducted from her total. Before response cost is introduced, you need to make sure your child is earning tokens and has "bought into" the token economy plan. Make sure that you see it as motivating and that your child sees it as fun. Otherwise, it will become a frustrating exercise to your child and therefore useless as a strategy.

Reward charts and token economies are good ways to help motivate children to take responsibility for their own behavioral improvement when praise alone has not been effective enough. They also help parents facilitate these gains in structured, positive, consistent, and objective ways. These techniques work especially well when the rewards for compliance are fairly immediate (getting the tokens as soon as possible after complying, and going on the earned and agreed-on trip to the beach within a week). Their effectiveness is also enhanced

EFFECTIVE BEHAVIORAL TECHNIQUES FOR CHILDREN WITH ATTENTION-DEFICIT/ HYPERACTIVITY DISORDER

Technique	Description	Example
Positive reinforcement	Providing rewards or privileges dependent on the child's performance.	Child completes an assignment and is permitted to play on the computer.
Ignoring behavior	In response to the child's unwanted behavior, parents do not pay attention to it—neither with their body language nor responding in words. They actively ignore it.	When the child recognizes that her negative behavior is not getting the attention she desires, she may first escalate the behavior (extinction burst), but when she sees that it never gets the attention she desires it will stop (extinguish).
Time-out	Removing access to positive reinforcement contingent on performance of unwanted or problem behavior.	Child hits sibling and, after ignoring the command to stop and being told the choices for complying or not complying, is required to sit for 5 minutes in the corner of the room.
Response cost	Withdrawing rewards or privileges contingent on the performance of unwanted or problem behavior.	Child loses free-time privileges for not completing homework by the indicated deadline.
Token economy	Child earns rewards and privileges contingent on performing desired behaviors. This type of positive reinforcement can be combined with response cost, where a child can also lose the rewards and privileges based on undesirable behavior.	Child earns stars for completing assignments and loses stars for getting out of seat. The child cashes in the sum of stars at the end of the week for a prize.

when your child gets the opportunity to help create the list of goals, the assigned value of each behavior, and the rewards that follow satisfactory compliance. It is also best to do what you can to keep point deductions to a minimum (by breaking tasks up into reasonable steps and not expecting too much too soon) so that your child does not become too discouraged and give up. Some children do not start to warm up to token economies until they have experienced one or more of the promised "big rewards," so be sure to continue the technique for 1 or more months—as long as your child does not become too frustrated or resistant—before deciding whether it is useful for her. Keeping her goals achievable and the program positive will go a long way toward making this approach successful.

Using Punishment Effectively

No one likes to invoke negative consequences for unacceptable behavior, but doing so calmly and consistently is a necessary part of helping your child learn new ways of functioning. At first it can be difficult to decide when punishment is appropriate because it is easy to attribute much of your child's failure to manage some of her behaviors appropriately to "her ADHD." Refusal to obey, when it does occur along with ADHD, can be greatly reduced with effective parenting techniques.

When parents think about "discipline" and punishment, they may think about spanking (without causing physical injury) as a way to reduce or stop undesirable behavior. Many studies have shown that spanking is, however, a less effective strategy than time-outs or removal of privileges for achieving these goals. In addition, spanking models aggressive behavior as a solution to conflict and can lead to agitated or aggressive behavior, physical injury, or resentment toward parents and deterioration of parent-child relationships. Most experts and organizations, including the AAP, discourage the use of spanking as a strategy for punishment. Spanking when a parent is out of control is considered physical abuse.

Time-outs and loss of privileges are the 2 forms of punishment that have been proven effective for children with ADHD. They are appropriate tools for responding to the few behaviors you have identified as intolerable. Time-outs, most often used with younger children, involve sending your child to a specified room (with no entertaining distractions and a door that can be closed) or chair (where you can see her) until the end of a preset time—

typically about 1 minute per year of the child's age (usually no longer than 5 minutes). Before instituting time-outs, you must discuss your intention with your child, explaining that they will be the consequences of violating the family's most important rules. Explain that unless behaviors are dangerous and need to be stopped right away, you will always give a terminating command ("Give your brother's toy back.") and a warning ("If you don't give it back within one minute you'll be in a time-out.") before you impose a time-out, so that your child will always be able to choose to avoid it by changing her behavior (making a good choice) on the spot. Keeping in mind the difficulty with time perception that some children with ADHD experience, tell your child that you will use a timer to measure the length of the time-out, and demonstrate to her how the timer works.

Once your child understands how time-outs work, you can begin to implement them when appropriate. When your child displays an unacceptable behavior

- Warn her that a time-out will occur if she does not respond to your warning in a specific amount of time ("Anna, stop pushing your sister. If you haven't stopped by the time I count to three, you will have a time-out.") or set number of prompts. Also state the consequences for choosing the appropriate behavior.

- If she does not comply in the specified time or number of prompts, firmly but calmly send her to the time-out setting. Do not give her more time to comply or let her engage you in any distracting interaction. Remember that she has made this choice herself by noncompliance.

- Tell her how many minutes the time-out will last, set a timer, and leave her alone—do not start negotiating whether she can get out earlier, or avoid going in. Another way to end a time-out is to wait until a child self-calms for 2 to 5 seconds. In this manner, the child learns that self-calming is what ends the time-out. Some experts suggest adding another minute to the time-out each time your child leaves the time-out space or is disruptive, then allowing her out at the end of that time if she is quiet and cooperative.

- When she has completed the time-out process, make a point of praising her next positive behavior so that the negative "punishment" experience is fully ended.

Be prepared for a great deal of resistance the first few times when time-outs occur. Soon, however, your child will learn that you are remaining consistent; that resisting, arguing, or negotiating no longer work; and that it is better to choose the positive behavior and avoid the time-out altogether. Meanwhile, remember that the goal is for your child to focus on staying out of time-outs rather than getting out of them once she has "chosen" to take the time-out rather than complying with your request to stop an unacceptable behavior. Remember also that a time-out is time out from "time-in"—meaning that the only reason your child will care if she gets a time-out is if she is used to loving, positive, and fun family interactions that will be missed during the time-out period. By supporting your child in these positive ways while sticking to the rules you have created, you can help your child learn to control her behavior and respect your fair and consistent requests and commands. An alternative to time-out for some children is "job grounding," where a child is grounded until a job that they select from a random list of jobs is successfully completed.

Loss of privileges, a more appropriate negative consequence for older children and teenagers, consists of invoking a "cost" for intolerable behavior. If your child breaks a family rule or ignores a command after a pre–agreed-on number of warnings, privileges are removed for a time appropriate to the seriousness of the transgression. This technique works best if your child has participated in decisions about exactly which behaviors will merit a loss of privileges and agrees in advance to some pre-negotiated penalties. It is also a good idea to try to relate the penalty as closely as possible to the transgression. Your child's failure to complete her homework, for example, may cost her television privileges the next day, while a teenager's failure to return home after curfew may cause her to lose car privileges for the weekend. These techniques do not work well when extensive consequences (3 weeks without driving or television) are imposed. After the immediate consequences for the inappropriate behavior there is no more learning value. Long consequences just foster resentment toward parents and become harder and harder to enforce, making them ineffective tools.

If you find that your child continues to strongly resist complying with time-outs or loss of privileges while continuing the negative behaviors, consider the way in which you are implementing these techniques. If you have been giving in to her resistance—allowing her out of the time-out area if she yells and kicks long enough, or letting her negotiate her way out of a loss-of-privilege punishment—she will have learned that resistance allows her to have her way. If you have been enforcing the rules sometimes, but not every time, she may not be able to resist testing your responses on every occasion to learn what you will do this time. If you have successfully carried out an effective punishment procedure but neglected to work on fostering a successful supportive, fun, and well-structured "time-in" home environment, your child may have decided she will never be able to succeed and give up trying. These are the reasons why it is so important to remain calm, firm, and consistent while invoking a punishment and to follow up as soon as possible with reassuring praise.

Managing Your Child's Behavior in Public

With proper training and practice, behavior therapy techniques can become relatively simple to implement at home, where a time-out area is clearly identified and it is possible to respond immediately to unacceptable behavior. Parents are often most disturbed by intolerable behavior when it occurs in public, however, because they feel that other adults—who do not know that their child has ADHD and have no idea how much progress she has already made—are negatively judging their child and their parenting skills. In any case, children with ADHD need to learn to manage their behavior wherever they are, so it is important to establish methods for implementing disciplinary techniques outside the home.

The most effective behavior management methods for use in public are the same ones you have developed with your child at home. If she is already familiar with the standard costs for certain types of behavior, you may need only remind her privately of the 2 or 3 main behavior rules she most needs to keep in mind before you enter the new environment, what positives will result from her following these rules, and what the cost will be for breaking them. To help her maintain her efforts to comply, praise her positive behaviors occasionally during the outing and let her know you appreciate how hard she is trying to follow the rules—that is, "catch her being good." If she manages to control her behavior throughout the entire period, acknowledge the difficulty of this feat and give her special praise. If you have also offered a reward, then provide it as soon as possible.

If your child refuses or fails to behave acceptably, even after a final warning, you will need to invoke the appropriate negative consequence. Do not delay just because you are among other people; such delay will probably just lead to increased misbehavior. You can enforce token economy "fines" or removal of privileges practically anywhere (as long as you keep your conversation private), but you may need to talk with your child's therapist ahead of time about how you might implement them discreetly yet effectively at the supermarket, your friend's house, church, or wherever you expect to be.

Your child needs your competent handling of rewards and limits as she practices new behavioral rules in public, but she also needs your thoughtful planning if she is to successfully

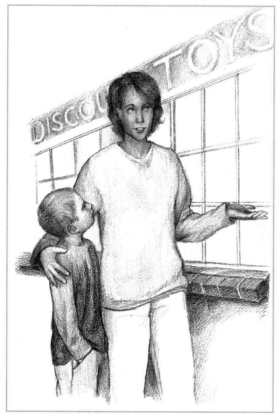

maintain her best self-control in these situations. Planning in advance can make all the difference in her ability to control her restlessness and stay focused. Whenever you take her along on errands, to a restaurant or friend's house, or for a trip—even across town—be sure to pack some activities to keep her happily occupied (activity books, handheld computer games, paper and pen). Once you are in public together, involve her in your activity if possible (helping choose items at the store, helping to make a snack at your friend's house).

Before entering a new environment, remind your child which 2 or 3 behavior rules he needs to follow. Praise his positive behaviors during the outing and let him know you appreciate how hard he is trying to follow the rules.

Maintaining the Gains From Parent Training After the Sessions Are Finished

Before your behavioral parent training program is complete, you should discuss ways in which you can continue to help your child work toward her targeted outcomes in the months and years to come. You will have learned how to recognize when a desired goal has been reasonably achieved and when and how to formulate new targets with your child, her teacher, and the rest of her treatment team. You should also discuss the ways in which you will need to adapt your parenting techniques to your growing child's new stages of development. While behavioral parent training programs do focus in large part on younger children, you will learn how to move from time-outs to response-cost techniques as your child grows, and to include her more and more in discussions about behavioral goals, rewards and punishments, and treatment decisions.

Making the Most Out of Parenting Techniques

Clearly, parent training and techniques take a great deal of effort on your part. It is always difficult to change old habits, and altering your parenting approach can be especially challenging because it often springs from what happened in your own family as you were growing up and your deep-seated childhood experiences. Being able to participate in a formal parent training program is an optimal way to learn, practice, and get feedback on the techniques discussed in this chapter, but if this is not possible for any number of reasons, you can also work on these principles with your child's pediatrician or psychologist in a less formal way. While reading this material can give you a general idea of how behavior therapy works, actually participating in parent training or working with professionals in other ways allows you to tailor its methods to your own unique situation, try out some of the techniques under expert guidance, and get regular feedback on what is and is not working and on how to adjust your approach. Without this focused support, you might find success more limited.

If you decide to look further into parent training, ask your pediatrician for a referral. As you read earlier, the focus of these parenting programs will be on helping you understand your child's ADHD behaviors, and teaching you skills to deal effectively with and help improve those behaviors. For example, you'll learn to effectively talk with him about his behavior and how to reinforce positive actions. Research has shown that parent training and classroom behavior interventions have been able to successfully change the behavior of children with ADHD.

Keep in mind, too, that behavior therapies, including parent training, have been shown to be effective only while they are being implemented and maintained. (Your child is not likely to keep up her improved behavior if you drop the effective techniques you have learned.) Even during periods when you see little progress, it is important to remain consistent. During those times when you feel exhausted and discouraged, and wonder what the point is of trying (and many parents of children with ADHD do get to that point once in a while), consider how hard your child must also work to continue trying to maintain her best self-control. By focusing as much as possible on the positive, thinking creatively, and asking for expert help when needed, you can maintain the supportive structure you have created for your child and eventually see measurable improvement. Sound programs also usually include support to help parents and children maintain the progress that's been made and prevent relapses. Similar to with medication, behavioral therapies are only effective while they are being implemented and maintained. Finally, parents need to take care of themselves if these or any other interventions are going to work well. Some factors that interfere the most with successful behavior therapy are maternal depression and maternal social isolation. Those parents who are having difficulty dealing with these issues in their own lives often benefit significantly from getting help for themselves, both in the form of cognitive-behavioral therapy and/or medication.

Additional Approaches

As noted previously, a variety of factors may limit the effectiveness of parent training in some circumstances. When ADHD is accompanied by oppositional defiant disorder, conduct disorder, and mood and anxiety disorders, these coexisting conditions can compound the behavioral challenges presented by children and adolescents with ADHD and can contribute to aggressive behavior, poor tolerance for frustration, inflexibility, poor problem-solving skills, heightened difficulty in complying with parents' instructions, and significant family conflict. When such conditions are present, additional treatment approaches may be useful.

One such model, developed by Dr Ross Greene, is called the collaborative problem-solving (CPS) approach. This cognitive-behavioral approach arises from some of the same theoretical underpinnings of parent training, but focuses more on helping adults and children become proficient at resolving problems collaboratively as a means of defusing conflict and teaching kids the cognitive skills they may lack. Through this joint approach, both parent and child learn to resolve issues in a mutually acceptable way.

According to this model, the manner in which adults solve problems with their children is a major factor influencing the frequency and intensity of oppositional outbursts. The CPS approach describes 3 basic options for solving the problems that are reliably and predictably precipitating adult-child conflict: (a) imposition of adult will (unilateral problem-solving), often accompanied by adult-imposed consequences; (b) collaborative problem-solving; and (c) deferring resolution of the problem, at least for now. Imposition of adult will is the most common cause of oppositional outbursts. Deferring resolution of a given problem removes low-priority adult expectations, at least temporarily, so that the adult and child can focus on higher-priority problems first. This option is effective at reducing tension between the child and parent and decreasing explosive outbursts. The second option, the proactive, collaborative resolution of problems, helps adults pursue their behavioral expectations without increasing the likelihood of oppositional outbursts. It also gives parents and children training and practice in regulating their emotions, dealing with frustration, and solving problems in a realistic and mutually satisfactory manner. Treatment sessions focus on helping children and adults successfully master the CPS approach.

Adults are viewed as the "facilitators" of the collaborative problem-solving process. In fact, adults are often told that their role is to (a) help their child reduce the likelihood of oppositional outbursts in the moment and (b) help their child develop skills to handle frustration and resolve problems over the longer term. Adults are helped to identify the specific "unsolved problems" that are reliably precipitating challenging episodes. Common unsolved problems include teeth brushing, getting to bed at night, waking up in the morning, homework, screen time, dietary choices, and sibling interactions. The process of identifying specific unsolved problems helps adults come to recognize that a child's challenging behavior is, in fact, highly predictable and that the problems setting the stage for the challenging behavior can be resolved proactively. Thus, rather than simply reacting to the outbursts by imposing consequences, parents are instead helped to resolve the problems giving rise to those outbursts. In other words, adults are strongly encouraged to adopt a "crisis prevention" mentality instead of a "crisis management" mentality. Adults are then helped to master the "ingredients" involved in solving problems collaboratively, including (1) achieving the clearest possible understanding of the child's concern or perspective on a given unsolved problem, (2) entering the adult's concern or perspective on the same unsolved problem into consideration, and (3) brainstorming solutions that are realistic and mutually satisfactory (meaning the concerns of both parties are addressed). The CPS approach differs from other anger management and problem-solving training programs in its emphasis on helping adults and children develop the skills to resolve disagreements collaboratively. The process of solving problems collaboratively can be applied right at the moment that the oppositional behavior is about to occur, but is far more effective when problems likely to precipitate oppositional episodes are resolved proactively, well in advance, and when all of the adults at home, and even teachers, are involved and trained. More information about this approach can be found at www.livesinthebalance.org. Other resources for information on behavior therapy are found in the Resources section or page 311.

You may hear or read of other behaviorally oriented treatments for ADHD. Some with limited or no evidence of effectiveness include cognitive-behavioral therapy (although this can be quite valuable for some of the coexisting conditions and shows a bit more promise for adolescents with ADHD), social skills training, insight-oriented psychotherapy, and play therapy. Other more alternative therapies, such as vestibular stimulation, biofeedback, relaxation training, electroencephalographic biofeedback, and sensory integration exercises, lack the sufficient scientific support needed to be recommend as effective treatments.

Remember that these behavioral treatments, just like medication management, are not curative. In addition, no one would claim that ADHD arises from faulty learning or that several months of contingency management would produce sustained benefits for children with ADHD once treatment is withdrawn. Behavioral methods are largely a method of rearranging environments by artificial means to yield improved participation in major life activities.

No matter what approach you ultimately use, seek the guidance of a professional specifically trained to provide effective behavioral therapies. Not all approaches sometimes recommended for ADHD are helpful for children with ADHD, including play therapy and talk therapy, which have not been shown to be effective in treating the core symptoms of this condition. Remember also that ADHD is a highly heritable condition, making it likely that one or both parents may also have some of the same difficulties as their child. Because of that, the successful outcomes for your child may be more difficult to achieve. Behavioral therapy techniques can also be more difficult to use if either parent is depressed, has other emotional or mental health problems, or is under undue stress. This is just a reminder that taking care of yourself and your needs is one of the primary considerations for helping your child.

Q & A

Q: *Our child's pediatrician has recommended parenting training classes for my husband and me as a part of our son's treatment for ADHD. We have read about some of the techniques used in behavior therapy and they seem much like what we have already implemented with our other children. Anyway, it seems to us that it's our child who needs therapy more than we do, because we are already pretty consistent and predictable in our parenting style. Wouldn't he benefit more from a therapist who could help him work on controlling his behavior and obeying commands?*

A: The parenting techniques taught in behavior therapy courses designed for families of children with ADHD are noticeably similar to the positive parenting practices used by many parents. However, parent training provides an opportunity to think about these techniques in the much more structured, detailed, and consistent ways necessary to help with behavior changes with your son, who is posing a much greater behavioral challenge for you than your other children. Parent training directly addresses the behaviors that need to be changed and gives you the tools to make those changes. There is generally a lack of literature establishing the effectiveness of treatments other than behavior therapy approaches with ADHD.

Q: *I have implemented a number of behavior therapy techniques, including time-outs, star rewards charts, and a token system, at home with my child. But I find that, while these techniques work well when I first use them, they tend to lose their effectiveness as time passes. Is it necessary to rotate various techniques, phasing in new ones as older ones become less useful?*

A: Many families do find that certain techniques seem less effective over time, whether this is due to a child's "growing out" of them (becoming too old for time-outs, for example), that certain rewards become boring, or for many other reasons. As with medication or any other part of your child's treatment plan, it is essential to monitor the effects of behavior therapy techniques on your child's functioning—and to alter the treatment if a particular technique is found not to be working. Your ongoing monitoring of how well your approach supports your child's functioning, and your willingness to change techniques to help your child, will not only help your family work more efficiently but will demonstrate to your child your concern for her well-being and involvement in her life. The principles that you have learned remain sound, although you may need to alter some of the details. Whenever possible, keep your child involved with making sure that the reward process remains fun and the consequences seem fair.

Q: *I have attended a behavior therapy course designed for parents of children with ADHD and have started using many of the techniques at home with some success. My problem, though, is that my son's father, from whom I'm divorced, refuses to learn about these techniques and use them when my son is with him. How can I maintain a structured life for my son when he is basically on his own every other weekend at his father's house?*

A: Separate households can present quite a challenge to families of children with ADHD because consistency is so important for the progress of these children. It is optimal to have your ex-spouse involved as much as possible from the very beginning of the evaluation through developing and carrying out a treatment plan. This will remain in the best interest of your child, and encourage their buy-in and cooperation with the treatment plan because their opinions have been respected, their questions answered, and their input sought as the plan develops. If a breakdown in communication remains, your child's pediatrician may be able to recommend a family therapist who can help you and your ex-spouse work through some of the issues that are standing in the way of a consistent routine that can be maintained in both households. If none of these possibilities are feasible, however, you should still implement and role model as many of these behavior therapy techniques as you can in your own household.

Chapter 7

Your Child at School

School can be particularly challenging for children with attention-deficit/hyperactivity disorder (ADHD), who often experience poor academic performance, behavior problems, and difficulties with social interaction. Coexisting conditions, such as a learning disability, an anxiety disorder, or disruptive behavior problems, can make it even more difficult for a child to succeed. The situation can be further complicated by the fact that there is no typical, predictable classroom style common to all children with ADHD—some parents

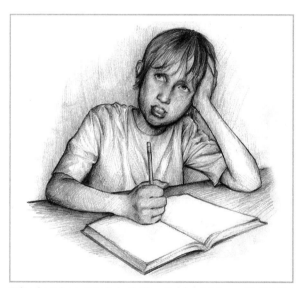

School can be particularly challenging for children with ADHD.

of children with ADHD may receive reports that their child is "not trying hard enough" academically, while others may be told that their child turns in acceptable work but frequently violates classroom rules. It can be hard for you as a parent to tell how much of any problem identified by a teacher falls into the normal range of child development, how much is due to ADHD, and how much is due to a coexisting problem (see Chapter 9). Add to this the fact that the focus of your child's problems may change from year to year—from largely behavioral to academic, from academic to social, and so on. It is small wonder that children with ADHD and their families often find school issues so central to their overall concerns.

The better informed you are as a family about the many ways in which ADHD may affect your child's school experience, the better prepared you will be to anticipate and deal with problems before they become insurmountable. You can use the information provided in this chapter to help foster your child's academic and social success in school. In the following pages, you will learn

- What types of school-related challenges children with ADHD face most often
- How to identify your own child's particular areas of concern
- Which classroom structures, school policies, teaching styles, and accommodations can best support your child's learning
- What an Individualized Education Program (IEP) is and how to work with your child, his teachers, and the school team to create one
- How to promote school success at home and elsewhere

What Types of Challenges Do Children With ADHD Typically Face at School?

Because ADHD can limit a child's ability to pay attention and control impulses and behavior, it is easy to imagine how problems in these areas can affect many aspects of school life, and how such problems can increase if not addressed effectively early on. In general, children with ADHD experience their greatest challenges in the areas of *behavior management, academic progress,* and *social interaction.* Due to changing school demands and changes in your child's symptoms, she may face greater problems in one area at a particular age and in another as she grows older. It is important to continue observing your child's functioning in each of these areas, and to encourage her to gain skills in monitoring her own functioning, to address any emerging problems as soon as possible.

Behavior Issues

Disruptive behavior is a common expression of hyperactive-impulsive– and combined-type ADHD, and can begin to create real problems as a child enters kindergarten or elementary school. Because so many of the demands in the early school years involve following rules and settling down, the inability to meet these demands is what frequently leads to questions about whether a child might have ADHD. A teacher may report that such a child "talks too much," "acts out constantly," or "doesn't seem to recognize limits." Teachers may suggest that the child's impulsive behavior is alienating the other children or making it difficult to maintain order in the classroom and on the playground. As a child with hyperactive-impulsive– or combined-type ADHD grows, the ADHD symptoms may begin to be expressed less in physical terms and more verbally. The child may interrupt frequently or speak out of turn, and perhaps even "mouth off" to authority figures or his classmates.

Other factors not directly attributable to ADHD may increase your child's behavior problems at school. Parents' or teachers' lack of knowledge about how to support or work with a child with ADHD, or a child's past negative preschool or child care experiences, can damage his self-esteem or attitude. This can cause him to give up trying to follow rules or please authority figures, at least temporarily. Coexisting conditions, such as depression, can also intensify a child's difficulties.

Even the normal developmental stages of childhood, such as a sixth-grader's testing of boundaries (refusing to do homework) or an adolescent's desire not to seem different from his classmates (avoiding taking medication), can have a negative effect on his functioning. Stresses in the home environment—marital conflict, financial difficulties, discipline problems, or other issues—can also affect your child's behavior at school. Finally, it is important to remember the role that general health plays in your child's behavior. Every child, including children with ADHD, should receive routine medical care and have his vision and hearing tested.

Academic Concerns

While behavior management issues are often the first school-related problems that children with ADHD experience, academic progress often becomes an area of increasing concern. Regardless of your child's intellectual abilities, she may find it hard to meet academic expectations as her symptoms interfere with her ability to learn, or she fails to receive some of the academic supports that she needs. Because it is difficult for many children with ADHD to stay on task and work independently for long periods, they often complete less work and thus have fewer chances to respond appropriately during the teacher's instruction. Problems with work production (incomplete work, sloppiness, failure to follow instructions) and inconsistency (satisfactory work one day and poor output the next) can become major barriers to school success. This may partially account for the estimates that 60% to 80% of children with ADHD underachieve academically and are identified by their teachers with some school performance problems. About 20% of children with ADHD have specific learning disabilities, such as a reading disorder, mathematics disorder, or expressive language disorder, that are separate from their ADHD symptoms (see Chapter 9).

It is easy to see how many ADHD-type behaviors can interfere with successful learning in a typical classroom. Your child's distractibility and lack of persistence may prevent her from retaining material taught in class. Her impulsivity may cause her to rush through schoolwork and respond spontaneously to questions instead of thinking ideas through. A poor sense of time, characteristic of many children with ADHD, can make long homework assignments, time-limited tasks, and test-taking extremely difficult. Organizing, planning, and sequencing problems lead to incomplete work, poor note-taking skills, or an inability to follow a work schedule or finish a long assignment. Poor fine motor planning can make the actual writing process difficult—limiting your child's ability to take notes, complete tests, and write effortlessly. Short-term memory problems can make it difficult to memorize facts. Inconsistencies and fluctuations in performance are common. Children with ADHD can also do well in any of these areas one day and poorly the next.

Around the fourth grade, as more academic focus and work production is required (as students move from "learning to read" to "reading to learn"), children with inattentive- or combined-type ADHD often begin to fall behind academically. Failure to pay attention to classroom lectures and turn in homework are typical symptoms that alert teachers to a child's difficulties.

As children with ADHD enter middle school and high school, they may encounter new challenges due to poor organizational skills, incomplete work, or a failure to turn work in. Because many of these behaviors are also experienced by children who do not have ADHD, your child's teacher may suggest that these problems are due to lack of motivation, low self-esteem, or other psychological causes. However, as you will read, when children with ADHD have these problems, they may qualify for extra support in school to help with overcoming or bypassing these obstacles. By middle school academic performance can also decline if medication schedules are not adjusted to cover lengthening homework time (in situations where medication is indicated and has been helpful), or if a child's treatment plan fails to meet her changing needs in other ways.

When a child is far behind in learning, a learning disability should be suspected. Children with coexisting learning disabilities may experience more long-lasting and serious academic difficulties than those struggling academically on the basis of ADHD alone. Learning disabilities are diagnosed when a child has not developed specific academic skills at the expected level in spite of adequate intelligence and education. The category of learning disabilities is designated by schools. Schools do not medically diagnose conditions, but rather determine if a child's apparent need, such as a learning problem, will qualify that child for special education services under a disability category, such as a specific learning disability. Federal legislation requires each state to develop its own criteria for determining a specific learning disability. The criteria must allow use of a process based on the child's response to scientific, research-based educational interventions. This is often called response to intervention or RTI. The category of specific learning disabilities is defined by federal definition as "a disorder in one or more of the basic psychological processes involved in understanding or in using language, spoken or written, that can result in the imperfect ability to listen, think, speak, read, write, spell, or do mathematical calculations."

A student with a learning disability in one area may excel in others. Some children with learning disabilities may have excellent verbal and reading skills, for example, but do poorly in math, while others may have the opposite profile. Keep in mind, however, that ADHD is not itself a learning disorder, that it does not *necessarily* lead to academic difficulties at school, and that neither ADHD nor learning disabilities are signs of low intelligence. In fact, children with ADHD display the same range of intelligence as their classmates. Learning disabilities are recognized in reading, mathematics, and written expression, and will be discussed in more detail in Chapter 9.

Social Concerns

For many children with ADHD, interactions with classmates tend to become difficult at one time or another. Children with ADHD can be disliked, ignored, or rejected by their peers. Some children with ADHD can be impulsive and intrusive in social relationships, physically or verbally overwhelming others. Others may not initiate interactions with their classmates, or miss the social cues necessary to establish positive relationships, and thus become socially isolated. Inattentiveness or impulsivity may decrease a child's success in games, sports, or other group activities that would otherwise enhance popularity. Younger children with hyperactive-impulsive– or combined-type ADHD may frequently experience physical conflicts with their peers, pushing their way into lines, or being "in their face." By middle childhood, a child's hyperactive-impulsive–type behaviors, discipline problems, perceived "spaciness," or social awkwardness may lead to social rejection. Some adolescents with ADHD may be 1 to 2 years less mature than their classmates, further complicating their social relationships at a time when they are taking on great importance.

Later in this chapter, you will find suggested ways for you and your child's teacher to provide opportunities for your child to improve her social standing and interact more successfully with her peers. Meanwhile, social concerns should be discussed at any meeting aimed at evaluating your child's progress and needs.

Beginning to Identify the Key Areas of Concern

Helping a child with ADHD to better manage his school life is best done in the same way you began to address his functioning in other areas, by

1. Identifying the greatest obstacles to his best functioning
2. Creating a treatment plan to address these concerns
3. Establishing a system of review aimed at measuring the treatment's success and failure and adjusting the plan appropriately

Because problems differ from one child with ADHD to the next, and even from one year to the next in a single child, academic, behavioral, and social functioning should all be reviewed carefully. Your greatest ally in arriving at an accurate assessment is your child's teacher because she observes your child in the classroom each day and can compare his functioning to that of his peers. A teacher's willingness to work with you, your child, and your child's pediatrician to meet your child's needs—and your own efforts to show an equal willingness to work through any differences of opinion to come up with an effective education program—can be an important factor in the extent of your child's success and failure in any given year.

The first step in improving your child's experience at school is to arrange to meet with his teacher to discuss his functioning and to listen carefully to the teacher's description of your child's school problems. If at all possible, bring your child with you for at least parts of this and any other parent-teacher meetings so that he can help clarify some of the observations and participate in generating ideas for resolving problems. His participation may add important insights about his functioning, and his buy-in to the education program is necessary for success. If you suspect that you may miss or misunderstand important information conveyed by the teacher because of an emotional response to what you are hearing, take a notebook to your meetings to write down what she says for later review. Bringing a friend or relative to take notes while you listen can also be helpful. Some teachers will also be comfortable if you ask to record the meeting.

The emphasis at these initial meetings should be on describing problem behaviors that are specific and that can be measured, not on generalities about your child's symptoms, feelings, or intent. If the teacher suggests, for example, that your child does not seem to be trying to succeed academically, ask for specific examples, as in, "Is some of his homework turned in, or none of it?" "Is schoolwork complete one day and incomplete the next, or is it always incomplete?" "Does my child ignore deskwork, or try but fail to finish it?" "Does my child seem to deliberately try to disrupt the class while others are working?" If the teacher is concerned that your child is having problems getting along with others, ask whether this is due to a tendency to physically overwhelm them; intrude verbally on their conversations; seem isolated or unengaged; or have trouble participating in games due to a lack of coordination, lack of focus, or inability to wait his turn. Ask how frequently each type of conflict happens. These types of specific, quantifiable observations are also necessary as a good baseline for monitoring changes over time, and can help in identifying necessary modifications in your child's treatment plan. Do not become concerned if your observations of your child differ from his teacher's. This is common and can lead to some good discussions about why behaviors may be seen as differing between home and school.

During your first meetings, you and his teacher may not be able to precisely define the problems or agree on solutions. What is more important at this early stage is to *establish a cooperative relationship* and a plan for systematically gathering and analyzing observations in the future. This will be easier if you can set aside any past negative relations with school personnel and start fresh with this new person. Because more and more educators are learning about ADHD and the best ways to manage it at school, this year's teacher may show more insight into what is causing your child's problem or suggest some practical responses that have not been tried before. The more clearly you demonstrate your willingness to cooperate and be a member of the "treatment team" the more positive and effective your partnership with the school may become. Problems in the home environment—marital conflict, financial difficulties, discipline problems, or other issues—can affect your child's functioning at school and should be mentioned with discretion in your meetings with his teacher so that you can together arrive at an accurate picture of the challenges that your child faces.

Choosing the Most Appropriate Classroom Setting

Because most children with ADHD experience difficulties meeting some of the academic, social, and behavioral expectations of schools, schools need to play a critical role in providing behavioral and academic support for them. Unless your child has especially severe disruptive behaviors accompanying her ADHD or is diagnosed with certain coexisting conditions or disabilities, her needs can probably best be met in a regular classroom with proper treatment and appropriate support from you and the teacher. In fact, federal law mandates that children with disabilities, including those with ADHD, must be educated alongside children without disabilities as long as the regular classroom meets their needs and allows them to make educational progress. Still, a number of factors within your child's regular classroom environment—its physical setup, the sense of community that the students feel, the special resources provided, the educational approach used, the compatibility of your child's and his teacher's personal styles and, most crucially, the experience and commitment of the teacher and other school personnel—can have a profound effect on your child's progress. If you are in a position to choose the school your child will attend, or at least have input into her teacher for the coming school year, thorough research and a well-informed choice can make a great deal of difference to you both.

Your Child's Classroom

"My son's first-grade teacher has had a lot of problems with his behavior," writes one parent of a child with ADHD. "He has a hard time sitting still and focusing on deskwork. The teacher has been talking with me about ways to help him get better at this skill, but I wonder if my son might be better off in a less-structured classroom where he does not have to sit still as much." Many parents of children with ADHD believe that a more free-flowing classroom environment may allow them to learn more effectively, in their own way. In some ways, it makes intuitive sense that a child who is not fettered by the constraints of a typically organized classroom will be able to make use of his own unique learning strengths and style at his own pace. In fact, studies have shown that the opposite is usually true: Children with ADHD often make significantly better progress when the classroom is thoughtfully structured—that is, in an organized setting with clear rules and limits; immediate, appropriate enforcement; and predictable routines. Traditional classroom seating arrangements (desks facing forward) often work better than open-plan designs (students seated around tables or desks arranged in a circle). This type of classroom environment can help to cut down on distractions, thus making it easier for a child to focus and receive and retain information. Like training wheels on a young child's bicycle, they provide the balance and stability that a child with ADHD may not be able to create on his own. Smaller class size can be another important element that can help prevent sensory overload and allow the teacher to provide the individual support your child needs. The smaller the class the better, in most cases, with no more than a few students who need special educational or behavioral services.

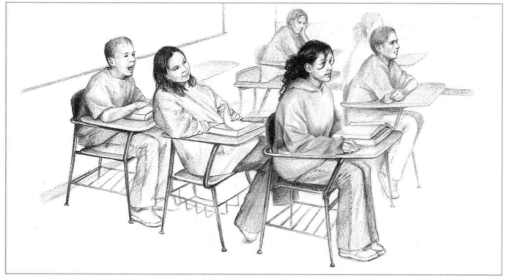

Traditional classroom seating (desks facing forward) can help to cut down on distractions, thus making it easier for your child to focus and receive and retain information.

The structure in a classroom can affect your child's day-to-day academic and social success. If frequent social conflicts are a problem during instruction time, it is easy to see how these may be avoided if students are seated facing the teacher instead of one another. If your child has trouble staying seated or remaining quiet when this is required, then clear limits and rules can be set with immediate positive feedback for following the rules and some consequences for noncompliance. It may also be possible to make some classroom accommodations. If your child has difficulty sticking to one task, frequent praise and encouragement when he is persistent may help extend his focus. Of course, just as with the behavior therapy parenting techniques you read about in Chapter 6, a structured environment works well only when it is designed to guide and support a child in positive ways rather than focusing on punishment and over-restriction. The thoughtfully structured routines of the ideal classroom environment should be balanced with a certain amount of variety, flexibility, and humor.

Your Child's Teacher

The most important member of your child's educational team is, of course, the teacher— particularly if your child will spend most or all of his time in a single classroom. The most effective teachers for children with ADHD are those who are generally informed and updated about it and the best ways to manage its related behavioral symptoms. If no such teacher is available, focus on requesting one with whom you feel comfortable and believe will be receptive to learning about ADHD from you, your child's pediatrician, and others. Training in and comfort using behavior management techniques should be a primary consideration. A natural, structured, and consistent teaching style is also a plus. Finally, teachers who speak expressively and who use a variety of different approaches (lectures, class discussion, audiovisual aids, computers) tend to engage the attention of a child with ADHD most successfully. A teacher who is structured and disciplined, but also dynamic, fun, and engaging, is the best choice for any student, including students with ADHD. If you have a chance to request a teacher for your child, it can help to ask older students and their parents for advice based on their experience. It can also help to make appointments to speak to prospective teachers about your child and your concerns, and to get a feel for their general teaching style and their working knowledge about students with ADHD. It is essential that you and the teacher feel comfortable exchanging ideas and planning strategies. You will spend a substantial amount of time together over the course of the school year. If possible, choose a teacher who is not only capable and knowledgeable, but with whom you feel you can connect. As you think about an ideal school environment outlined in this section, it may occur to you that, in many ways, your thoughts are similar to what every parent wants for his or her child.

- Small class size
- Regular routines
- A teacher who is engaging, interesting, fun, and exciting; who provides a great deal of structure but can also be flexible; and who is able and willing to use multiple approaches to teaching

It may help to remind yourself as you visit schools and talk with teachers that you are looking for what would be best for any student—but that this environment will be especially important for your child with ADHD.

Special Education Services—Federal Laws

For most children with ADHD, staying in a regular classroom with an excellent teacher, trained in and adept at behavior management, is the preferred situation. This is especially true if any necessary accommodations for your child can be put into place in that setting. Children with ADHD whose academic or behavior struggles cannot be managed effectively in a regular classroom using typical strategies may require special education services. These services may be delivered in a variety of settings, including the regular classroom and separate classrooms for part or all of a school day. The setting is determined by the needs of the eligible child. The federal law Individuals with Disabilities Education Act (IDEA) guarantees your child's right to be evaluated for and receive such services if eligible, free of charge.

IDEA

The IDEA was designed to guarantee the provision of special services for children whose disabilities severely affect their educational performance. A child can receive services under IDEA if she is learning disabled, emotionally disturbed, or "other health impaired." Your child may qualify for IDEA coverage if she has been diagnosed with ADHD and her condition has been shown to severely and adversely affect school performance. Note that both conditions must be met: an ADHD diagnosis alone does not guarantee coverage for your child unless it or another disorder is adversely affecting her educational performance. In most cases, it is a child's coexisting learning, disruptive behavior, anxiety, or other functional problem—not the ADHD itself—that qualifies her for IDEA coverage.

The IDEA is based on providing services for categories of disability. It includes 13 categories that require coverage "without undue delay." Under this law, schools are responsible for identifying and evaluating children who are suspected of having disabilities and who may need special education services. Depending on her diagnoses and assessment, your child's disability may be categorized as "specific learning disability," "serious emotional disturbance," or "other health impairment." After these needs are evaluated, documented, and eligibility determined, an IEP can be created to detail the special education services that are necessary.

Specific Learning Disabilities

The IDEA criteria for specific learning disabilities can vary from state to state. Children qualify for learning disabilities under this law if they have significant needs in the areas of

- Oral expression
- Listening comprehension
- Written expression
- Basic reading skills
- Reading comprehension
- Mathematics calculation
- Mathematics reasoning

Testing for learning disabilities generally includes assessment by the school psychologist.

In addition to learning disabilities, children with ADHD and significant emotional problems can also receive services through IDEA. To receive these services, a child's *educational performance* needs to be adversely affected by emotional and behavioral concerns:

- An inability to learn that can be best explained on a behavioral basis
- An inability to build or maintain relationships with peers and teachers
- Inappropriate types of behavior or feelings
- A persistent mood of unhappiness or depression
- A tendency to develop physical symptoms or fears associated with personal or school problems

A comprehensive evaluation that meets federal and state guidelines needs to be completed before children can qualify for services as emotionally disturbed. A note from your child's pediatrician that your child has ADHD or is depressed or anxious will not be enough to qualify her for services.

All children, including those with ADHD, are also eligible for services if they have the disabilities below and can be shown to need special education in order to benefit from their educational program.

- Intellectual or cognitive disabilities
- Hearing impairment, including deafness
- Speech or language impairment
- Visual impairment, including blindness
- Serious emotional disturbance
- Orthopedic impairment
- Autism spectrum disorders
- Traumatic brain injury
- Other health impairment, including ADHD and Tourette disorder
- Specific learning disabilities
- Developmental delay (used in some states for children aged 3–9 who have problems with development of their physical, cognitive, communication, social/emotional, or adaptive skills [everyday life skills]).

Additional considerations for eligibility include (1) schools cannot be overidentifying children in terms of race or ethnicity; (2) a child is not eligible for special education solely because of lack of instruction in academic areas; and (3) in newer IDEA legislation, children no longer need to demonstrate a severe discrepancy between their ability (IQ) and their achievement.

An alternative way to assess a child's need for special services, as mentioned previously, is RTI, an approach where a student with academic delays is given one or more research-validated interventions. The student's academic progress is monitored frequently to see if those interventions are sufficient to help the student catch up with his or her peers. If the student fails to show significantly improved academic skills despite several well-designed and implemented interventions, this failure to "respond to intervention" can be viewed as evidence of an underlying learning disability. One advantage of RTI in the diagnosis of educational disabilities is that it allows schools to intervene early to meet the needs of struggling learners and not require them to fail before anything is done.

"Other Health Impaired"

To qualify for services under "other health impaired," a child with ADHD needs to be documented as showing "limited strength, vitality, or alertness" that results in limited alertness in the educational environment, which adversely affects the child's educational performance. Attention-deficit/hyperactivity disorder is listed as one of the "chronic or acute health problems" that may lead to other health impairment eligibility.

IEPs

You as a parent can initiate a referral process if your child is doing poorly in academic, behavioral, or social functioning. The best way to make a referral is to write a letter to the principal outlining your concerns and requesting an evaluation. Send copies to your child's pediatrician as well as the school system's director of special education. The school will set up a meeting that must include you, the parents, to discuss the referral. Parents must always be included and involved in the identification and evaluation planning for their children. This group may plan the comprehensive evaluation at this meeting. Or this group may decide to try some accommodations or modifications in the regular education classroom before recommending a more comprehensive evaluation. Sometimes called pre-referral interventions, this may include RTI methods mentioned earlier.

The law states that a group of professionals from different disciplines must take part in the evaluation, and that it needs to be comprehensive and objective. Typical evaluations include

- Assessing your child using reliable, valid, individually administered tests
- Reviewing teachers' and parents' written observations
- Comparing your child's progress to that of others her age
- Interviewing you, the child, her teacher, and others who know or have worked with her

As a parent, you need to give informed consent before any evaluation is done. Keep in mind that the team is not required to accept a diagnosis that is made by an outside pediatrician or psychologist, and they may find a child ineligible for services. The decision must be justified by an evaluation, not just someone's opinion, and you have the right to dispute the decision.

An IEP That Meets Your Child's Unique Needs

After the evaluation has been completed, you must receive a written copy of the results, and you should meet with the evaluation team to discuss the results in detail. If the team determines that your child is eligible for special services under IDEA, then the team will develop an IEP. The IEP needs to meet your child's unique educational needs in the academic, behavioral, or social areas, and will go into effect once you sign it and agree to the program. The IEP will

- Address your child's present academic achievement and functional performance and how her disability affects her involvement and progress in the general curriculum.
- State all the supports to be provided, including special education, related services (such as counseling or occupational therapy), and any modifications.
- Set yearly measurable goals.
- Describe how and how often your child's progress on the goals will be measured.
- Explain any exceptions to a child participating with children in her regular class and in other school activities.
- Describe any necessary test-taking accommodations.
- Describe in detail when, where, and how often services will be provided.

Your child is entitled to an IEP that meets her unique educational needs. Her IEP may call for adjustments within the regular classroom, such as a structured learning environment; individualized test-taking conditions; the use of a tape recorder or computer; modified textbooks; individualized homework assignments; modifications during nonacademic times, such as lunchtime or recess; or other accommodations. It may call for the use of a classroom aide or note-taker, a trained tutor, or psychological or speech and language services. If your child's educational needs cannot be met through a regular classroom with these special supports, a self-contained special education classroom for part or all of a day may be proposed. After an IEP is written, then the special education team, which includes the parents, will meet at least once a year to see if the IEP needs to be modified. They can meet more often if the program requires changes based on how well or poorly certain approaches work for her. If the school no longer thinks that she needs these services, they need to reevaluate her to see if she still requires special education services. If her IEP is still in place during her high school years, then the team will also create a transition program to help with college, career, and/or daily living skills planning.

If you and the school district disagree at any point in the process about the request for an evaluation, the evaluation itself, or the resulting determination of the services needed, a variety of methods for dispute resolution are available in each state. As a parent, you can always contact your state's Department of Education for more details on this. Schools are also required to provide information on due process and parent rights.

Section 504

If your child does not qualify for services under IDEA, he may still qualify for services under Section 504 of the Rehabilitation Act, which prohibits discrimination against any person with a disability. Section 504, a civil rights law, applies to all public and private schools that receive federal financial assistance and is aimed at preventing discrimination against students with disabilities.

An important aspect of Section 504 is its emphasis on accommodating students with disabilities in *the regular classroom* whenever possible. This is done to help ensure that students with disabilities receive the same education as those without disabilities, while benefiting from whatever in-class accommodations are deemed necessary. Under Section 504 students may receive accommodations such as

- Reduced class size
- Preferential seating
- Modifications in homework and classroom assignments
- Extended time for testing
- Written instructions to supplement teachers' verbal instructions
- Behavior management strategies
- Help with organizing
- Note-takers

CHILDREN WITH DISABILITIES

Criteria for Section 504 Eligibility

Students with disabilities are defined in Section 504 as those who

- **Have a physical or mental impairment that substantially limits one or more "major life activities."** Because learning is considered a "major life activity," children who have been diagnosed with ADHD and who have significant difficulty learning in school are considered disabled under this law.

An evaluation is required to determine eligibility under Section 504. An eligible child may receive accommodations or modifications that are not available to nondisabled children. Children eligible for services under IDEA are also covered under Section 504, but the reverse is not true. Children covered by IDEA have a right to receive "educational benefit" while those covered under Section 504 are only protected from discrimination based on their disability. They have a right to access the same education as all children.

IDEA OR SECTION 504: WHICH IS MOST APPROPRIATE FOR YOUR CHILD?

The laws and regulations relating to ADHD can be confusing, and parents often aren't sure which is more beneficial for their child: to receive an IEP under IDEA or a Section 504 accommodation plan. It is the school district's evaluation that determines if a student is eligible under either IDEA or Section 504 for any such services or supports.

To qualify under IDEA, it must be determined that the disability is causing an adverse effect on the child's educational performance to the extent that special education is needed. If your child with ADHD has significant school difficulties, the provisions under IDEA have the following advantages:

- It provides for an individualized program tailored to meet the unique needs of the student.

- A wide range of program options, services, and supports is available.

- It sets out specific, measurable goals that are regularly monitored for progress.

- It provides funding for programs and services (Section 504 does not).

- It provides more protections with regard to the evaluation, how often reviews are done, parent participation, disciplinary actions, and other factors.

Section 504 plans serve many students well. For those students who qualify for a 504 plan, it is a faster and easier procedure for obtaining accommodations and supports (which may include some services). It may be more appropriate for

- Students with milder impairments who do not need special education
- Students whose educational needs can be addressed through adjustments, modifications, and accommodations in the general curriculum and classroom

---

Modified from: Rief S. *The ADD/ADHD Checklist: A Practical Reference for Parents & Teachers.* 2nd ed. 2008. This material is used by permission of Jossey-Bass, a Wiley Imprint.

In most cases, you will find that as a parent you are the driving force behind the evaluation process, and you may need to actively advocate for your child if he is to receive the services he needs. Parent support associations have made a great deal of progress in persuading states to follow federal guidelines, but cost considerations and lack of understanding of ADHD can limit a district's response. To learn about the federal, state, and local district guidelines regarding the services available to your child, contact your school district and your local chapter of Children and Adults With Attention-Deficit/Hyperactivity Disorder (CHADD), and consult the CHADD Web site and other sources of ADHD-linked support (see Resources on page 311).

What Can Schools Do?

General Classroom Supports

Earlier in this chapter you learned that certain aspects of your child's school environment, such as a structured routine and a traditional seating arrangement, can affect her ability to function. Other environment-related strategies shown to help children with ADHD include seating the child near the teacher and away from distractions, such as the windows, hallway, or pencil sharpener, and surrounding her with students who focus well on their own work. The teacher may even decide to create a "buddy system" for your child or for the class as a whole, in which children remind one another of academic, behavioral, or social goals and where the class as a whole earns points or tokens that can be traded in for privileges, like a class party. The less distracting your child's teacher can make your child's environment, the more likely it is that she will focus better on the task at hand. This way of preventing negative behavior from occurring in the first place is far preferable to trying to "fix" it later.

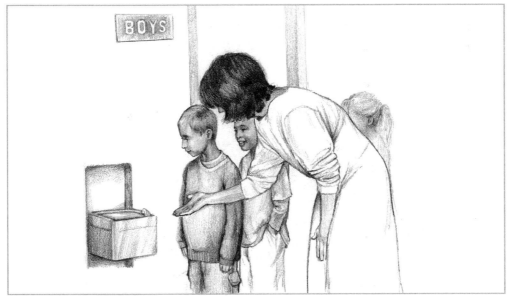

A simple routine, such as counting to 5 while taking a drink from the water fountain, may keep your child from getting distracted and playing.

HELPFUL TEACHER SUPPORTS FOR STUDENTS WITH ADHD

Keeping Things Simple and Doable
- Break down complicated instructions into doable steps.
- Adjust the length of assignments to fit a student's attention span.
- Keep the more academic subjects in the morning, when children are fresher and more alert.

Keeping Things Interesting
- Teach with enthusiasm and invite class participation.
- Vary lectures with hands-on experiences and physical activities.
- Supplement lectures with drills and computer games that teach the same materials to keep things novel, engaging, and motivating.

Keeping Things Organized
- Clearly state, repeat, and post the classroom rules. It is important for teachers to reinforce following classroom rules by regularly praising students who are complying.
- Preview the school day with a morning class meeting.
- Write things down for students who may miss verbal instructions or have trouble copying from the chalkboard.
- Encourage the use of simple daily planners that do not overwhelm students.

Your teacher will benefit from keeping the following mantra in mind as she works with your child in the classroom: *Keep things simple and doable, keep them interesting, and keep them well structured and organized. Emphasize the positive things that students are doing.*

As you have seen, most methods your child's teacher can implement are likely to benefit all of her students, not just your child. Nearly all children, by nature, are distractible and have problems with organization and staying focused at one time or another, and your child's peers will profit from the teacher's efforts to overcome this.

Schools and Behavior

Teachers, who must constantly deal with behavior problems in their classrooms, are generally encouraged to try prevention first, rewards for positive behavior second, and discipline measures only as a final resort when managing problem behaviors in any student. When teachers take this approach there is usually a dramatic improvement in how well the classroom functions and a noticeable reduction in how much classroom time is taken up with disciplinary measures. For children with ADHD and behavior concerns, IDEA actually mandates that the IEP team includes positive behavior approaches in the child's educational program.

Functional Behavior Assessments and Individual Behavior Plans

If the positive behavioral approaches described previously have proven unsuccessful, then a "functional behavior assessment" should be done. Functional assessments include a description of the behavior problems, direct observations of your child in different settings, and positive strategies to gradually decrease the specified behavior and increase other behaviors that are appropriate. Functional assessments are generally done by the school behavior specialist, who analyzes the triggers for specific problem behaviors, the behaviors that arise, and the consequences that are in place when those behaviors occur. The information is then used to try to understand the function of the behavior. For example, if a student gets out of his seat frequently and this disrupts the class, a functional analysis can help to pinpoint the reason—is it to avoid finishing an assignment or otherwise escape a situation? …to get attention?…to get something that he needs?…to create some self-stimulation in a quiet classroom? Each of these reasons may have different solutions, and a one-size-fits-all approach is inappropriate. The value of a functional analysis is that it can lead to a specific plan for your child's individual needs. Once this analysis is done, then this type of positive individualized plan can be created. A typical plan may include instituting preventive measures, teaching the child new behavior strategies, and using behavior therapy techniques to help him improve his functioning.

Preventive measures include changes that the teacher can make in the classroom environment to help students with ADHD avoid targeted behaviors. These include measures such as changing the seating arrangement in the classroom, altering classroom routines, posting the 5 most important classroom behavior rules on the chalkboard, or allowing frequent breaks during long assignments.

WHEN DISCIPLINE IS AN ISSUE

Many parents of children with ADHD feel that disciplinary actions tend to target their children due to a lack of understanding of ADHD-type behavior and reluctance to make appropriate accommodations and allowances. Children with serious behavior problems, such as extreme impulsiveness or a conduct disorder, may find themselves suspended from school over and over again while their behavior goes untreated.

Children covered under IDEA are protected to a large degree from such nonproductive disciplinary actions. Under the IDEA provisions, any child who has been identified as having a disability, who has demonstrated a need for services, or whose parents or teacher have expressed concern in writing or requested an evaluation may not be suspended or expelled for more than 10 consecutive days for behavior that is related to his disability. To determine whether the disability is a factor, the student's evaluation team, which includes his parents, must determine whether the conduct in question was caused by or had a direct relation to the child's disability or if the conduct was a direct result of the school's failure to implement the IEP. If the student's disability is determined to have been a factor or the IEP was not appropriately implemented, the child cannot be held to the same standards and arbitrarily suspended or reassigned to another program. Instead the child must be returned to his placement and a functional behavior assessment conducted or the current behavior plan modified to prevent similar behavior problems in the future.

Children covered under Section 504 are not as well protected. Section 504 does not require the school to keep the child in school or in ongoing programs while a reassessment takes place.

Students with ADHD can also be taught new strategies to replace their problem behaviors. For example, if your child disrupts the class during long assignments, a teacher might arrange a "secret signal" that he can use to let her know that he needs a break. When the teacher sees the signal she can respond by asking him to do a task that involves getting up and walking around.

The plan can also include teachers using the same behavior therapy principles that are taught in parent training. Techniques that have been found to be most successful in the classroom include

- Clearly conveying and consistently enforcing class rules
- Giving clear, doable commands
- Establishing daily goals for the child, and for the class as a whole
- Praising students for positive behaviors and ignoring negative behaviors that are not intolerable
- Using rewards to encourage appropriate behavior, which includes using token economies (point, sticker, and poker chip reward systems) and response-cost systems (losing tokens for inappropriate behaviors)
- Using appropriate nonphysical punishments, such as time-out to cut back on unacceptable behaviors
- Using behavior report cards to motivate children and enhance parent-teacher communication

The use of these techniques can not only help your child, but all the other children in the classroom as well. Regular communication between parents and teachers is essential to make some of these measures as effective as possible. A good working relationship with your child's teacher and the development of mutual respect will set a good tone for a team approach. For example, tokens earned in the classroom can be converted into rewards at home if there is good communication between parents and teachers.

Ideally, your child's teacher has received training in classroom behavior therapy techniques. In some, but not all, areas of the country, more teachers are trained in behavior therapy now than ever before. If your child's teacher has not received training, you may be able to advocate for teacher training funds, especially if you have requested services for your child under IDEA or Section 504 legislation. However, limited funding and support for such training means that your child's teacher may have to seek some of this information on her own. If you have participated in parent training, you and your trainer may be valuable resources. You may want to share any teaching materials and workbooks you used. There are also self-monitoring and self-evaluation strategies that children and adolescents can use. The CHADD Web site (www.chadd.org) and books that specifically address classroom intervention and school behavior therapy training programs (see the Resources section on page 311) are other good sources of information for teachers. Local ADHD support groups and other community resources may be helpful as well.

ADHD and Academics

Even if your child does not have a learning disability, the academic side of school can be difficult for students with ADHD. Some common concerns and practical suggestions are listed in the table on page 163.

Additional ideas for promoting academic success are available through some of the references in the Resources section on page 311.

The Social Side of School

Social difficulties are an aspect of school life that can become especially painful for a child with ADHD. Your child may have difficulty forming friendships due to a tendency to act before thinking, disruptiveness, failure to make plans, or acting inappropriately in spite of knowing what she is supposed to do. Children with inattentive-type ADHD often tend to be socially isolated or withdrawn. If you are concerned about your child's social experiences at school, talk with her teacher about ways to bolster her social confidence, increase her status, and help her improve her skills. If improvement in specific social skills is already part of her IEP or other education program, you and the teacher may already have brainstormed about behavior therapy techniques to reinforce and build on her skills in this area. Sound behavior management and medication approaches can go a long way toward improving the social functioning of children with ADHD. You might also suggest to the teacher such actions as casually but publicly praising your child for her talents or choosing her for classroom duties in front of other children. This allows other children to see her in a positive light and can enhance her self-esteem and sense of acceptance. You can also ask her teacher to intervene in tactful ways when she begins to fall into social difficulty and to find ways to set social skills goals, monitor her progress, and set up a system of rewards and privileges to recognize her for meeting her goals. Your child and her classmates might also benefit from class discussions about how we all manage our feelings, the value of diversity, and the importance of respect. It is surprising how effective a well-timed word or action can be.

ADHD AND ACADEMICS	
Area of Academic Difficulty	**Suggestions**
Written Expression *Difficulty with* • Fine motor skills • Attending to all aspects of written language at the same time • Following multiple or sequential steps (as in spelling) • Writing (considers it boring)	• Stimulant medications can sometimes markedly help fine motor paper and pencil skills. • Students with ADHD can start instruction in word processing by third grade and be permitted to complete assignments by computer.
Note-Taking *Difficulty with* • Listening and taking notes at the same time	• Teachers can provide students with lecture outlines or notes. • Students can listen to lectures and borrow a classmate's notes to study. • Students can tape-record lectures, but this can become tedious and time-consuming.
Rote Memorization Tasks • Requires sustained attention to tasks that are frequently boring	• Computer software can be a helpful and motivating way to memorize material like math facts.
Variations in Performance • Can occur from day to day or one grading period to the next	• Token economies and reward systems can help with motivation.

ADHD AND ACADEMICS (CONTINUED)	

Incomplete Assignments
 	
Can occur from
• Problems in following multiple directions
• Becoming bored with an assignment
	• The use of study cubicles has not been found to be helpful in increasing attention or concentration
	  – Computer-assisted instruction may be more stimulating and interesting and thus children may be more likely to complete an assignment that is computer-based, particularly in the context of educational game software (eg, "Math Blaster").
	• Classroom seating next to a positive peer model can lead to fewer off-task behaviors and greater work productivity.
	  – Peer tutoring can also be effective in helping students to practice academic skills.
	• In-school solutions should be found for incomplete classroom work, and teachers should avoid sending it home.

Organizational and Study Skills • Lost books • Assignments not turned in even if they have been completed • Messy and illegible papers	• Step-by-step tutoring on how to complete daily assignments and long-term projects. • Extra set of books at home. • Setting of homework time limits. • Modifications in homework assignments.
Reading Comprehension • Tuning out or getting distracted while reading	• Brief exercise breaks. • Parent reads part of the material while the child listens. • Parent and child discuss the material before, during, and after the material is read. • Older students preview the questions at the end of the chapter before reading the chapter so that they can focus on the most important points.

Modified from: Hannah JN. The role of schools in attention deficit hyperactivity disorder. *Pediatr Ann.* 2002;31:510. Originally printed in Hannah JN. *Parenting a Child With Attention Deficit Hyperactivity Disorder.* Austin, TX: Pro-ed; 1999. Used with permission.

If your school offers social-skills training groups, consider enrolling your child. Although effective social-skills treatments have been difficult to develop, programs in school with the classmates that your child interacts with every day are more likely to be successful than those run in clinics or other settings outside of school. Some of the most effective programs incorporate parents and teachers, help children to be aware of and understand verbal and nonverbal social cues, and use the same types of well thought out reward and response-cost systems that you read about in Chapter 6. They teach socially significant skills like good sportsmanship, problem-solving, accepting consequences, being assertive without being aggressive, ignoring classmates when they are provocative, and recognizing and dealing with feelings. In the better programs children are coached and receive feedback, and techniques are taught by role-playing real-life situations and modeling by coaches and teachers, and children receive reinforcement in real-world settings that they have learned as part of training. These types of programs can be incorporated into IEPs and behavior plans.

Closing the Gap Between Home and School

Daily Report Cards

Constant feedback for your child and frequent communication between you and her teacher are necessary components in keeping your child on track, and can make an enormous difference in how quickly positive results are seen. Both of these aims can be accomplished through daily report cards filled out by teachers and/or a journal for teachers' and parents' comments that your child keeps in her school backpack. A daily report card is especially effective because it identifies daily goals for your child, lets her see almost immediately how effectively she has met them, and motivates her to try harder to meet her goals as she receives agreed-on rewards for good reports. You and your child's teacher may find that it is best for you to provide some of these rewards at home because providing them in class takes up valuable class time, and some of the most effective rewards (such as telephone or television time) or negative consequences (such as restriction of privileges) may not be possible at school. Your willingness to respond appropriately at home can ease the teacher's workload and increase his willingness to work more closely with your child. Home-based reinforcements also highlight for your child the link between behavior at school and at home.

To develop this type of report card, you and your child's teachers first need to select the areas for improvement. A limited number of targeted behavioral or academic goals should be described as specifically as possible—in ways that are countable or measurable ("completes at least 80% of her worksheet during third period" not "stays on task"). These goals can then be translated into items to be checked off on the daily report that your child brings

SAMPLE DAILY REPORT CARD

Child's name: _____   Date: _____

	Special	Language Arts	Math	Reading	SS/ Science
Follows class rules with no more than 3 rule violations per period.	Y N	Y N	Y N	Y N	Y N
Completes assignments within the designated time.	Y N	Y N	Y N	Y N	Y N
Completes assignments at 80% accuracy.	Y N	Y N	Y N	Y N	Y N
Complies with teacher requests (no more than 3 instances of noncompliance per period).	Y N	Y N	Y N	Y N	Y N
No more than 3 instances of teasing per period.	Y N	Y N	Y N	Y N	Y N
Other					
Follows lunch rules.	Y N				
Follows recess rules.	Y N				

Total Number of Yeses: _____   Teacher's Initials: _____

Total Number of Nos: _____   Comments: _____

Percentage: _____   _____

Adapted with permission from: William E. Pelham Jr, PhD. School-Home Daily Report Card packet available for downloading at no cost at http://ccf.buffalo.edu.

home from school. Before using the report card system, arrange for a meeting including you, your child, and her teacher at which the process will be explained to your child, with a home-based reward system also set up to motivate her. At regular parent-teacher meetings throughout the school year, you can use the accumulated report cards to monitor your child's progress in accomplishing each task and modify items on the card when necessary. For more information about setting up a daily school-home report card, check the Comprehensive Treatment for Attention Deficit Disorder (CTADD) Web site (see the Resources section on page 311). A sample daily report card is provided on page 166. You can adapt this form to suit your child's targeted behaviors and the number of teachers she has. Again, the more precise and quantitative teachers can be when giving feedback, the more effectively these daily reports can be used to improve your child's education program.

Your child's teachers can record more detailed observations or requests in a journal that your child carries with her between home and school. You can also use the journal to inform a teacher of the behavior modification reward or cost your child received for her school performance. (For more information on reward-cost systems, see Chapter 6.) Daily report cards and a shared journal are efficient ways to keep in touch without having to constantly schedule meetings. They can also help your child keep her goals in mind and include her more in her own education program.

Ideally, this system of continuous communication will foster a positive working relationship between you and the teacher that can help your child achieve her goals. You may find, however, that you disagree with the teacher's approach or feel in conflict in some other way. If you have tried and failed to work productively as a team, consider asking your partner, the school principal or counselor, or even your child's pediatrician or therapist to mediate. Some local parent advocacy groups provide staff members to accompany parents to the school and help advocate for services. Your child's pediatrician or therapist may be able to help you locate this type of support. However, you will need to weigh the potential benefits of these types of actions against the possibility that the teacher may begin to see you as an adversary rather than a teammate—a position that will diminish your ability to advocate for your child. To help avoid such conflicts before they happen, be sure to express support for the teacher and help him in any way you can. If you are pleased with some aspects of his work, tell him and his principal. Your positive attention to the teacher will usually translate into positive attention to your child.

Homework

"I can't wait for summer to come!" writes the mother of a seventh-grader. "Suddenly the gloom lifts, the arguing stops, we relax, and we remember how much fun our family can have together." Dealing with issues around homework can be one of the most stressful and time-consuming elements of parenting in the family of a child with ADHD. Successfully dealing with homework production involves developing skills in time management, organization, and study habits; using behavior management techniques; and understanding your child's limits and frustration tolerance. Some hints are included in the Homework Tips for Parents box, and additional ideas are available in the Resources section on page 311.

HOMEWORK TIPS FOR PARENTS

- Establish a routine and schedule for homework (a specific time and place), and adhere to the schedule as closely as possible. Try not to have your child wait until the evening to get started.

- Limit distractions in the home during homework hours (reduce unnecessary noise, activity, and phone calls; turn off the television).

- Assist your child in dividing assignments into smaller parts or segments that are more manageable and less overwhelming.

- Assist your child in getting started on assignments (read the directions together, do the first items together, observe as your child does the next problem/item on his or her own). Then get up and leave.

- Monitor and give feedback without doing all the work together. You want your child to attempt as much as possible independently.

- Praise and compliment your child in a supportive, noncritical manner when he or she puts forth good effort and completes tasks.

- It is appropriate to assist in pointing out and making some corrections of errors on the homework.

- It is not your responsibility to correct all of your child's errors on homework or make him or her complete and turn in a perfect paper.

- Remind your child to do homework and offer incentives: "When you finish your homework, you can...."

HOMEWORK TIPS FOR PARENTS

- A contract for a larger incentive/reinforcer may be worked out as part of a plan to motivate your child to persist and follow through with homework: "If you have no missing or late homework assignments this next week, you will earn...."

- Let the teacher know your child's frustration and tolerance level in the evening. The teacher needs to be aware of the amount of time it takes your child to complete tasks and what efforts you are making to help at home.

- Help your child study for tests. Study together. Quiz your child in a variety of formats.

- If your child struggles with reading, help by reading the material together or reading it to your son or daughter.

- Work a certain amount of time and then stop working on homework. Do not force your child to spend an excessive and inappropriate amount of time on homework. If you feel your child worked enough for one night, write a note to the teacher attached to the homework.

- It is very common for students with ADHD to fail to turn in their finished work. It is very frustrating to know your child struggled to do the work, but then never gets credit for having done it. Papers seem to mysteriously vanish off the face of the earth! Supervise to make sure that completed work leaves the home and is in the notebook/backpack. You may want to arrange with the teacher a system for collecting the work immediately on arrival at school. E-mailing homework to the teacher is also helpful.

- Many parents find it very difficult to help their own child with schoolwork. Find someone who can. Consider hiring a tutor! Often a junior or senior high school student is ideal, depending on the needs and age of your child.

- Make sure your child has the phone number of a study buddy—at least one responsible classmate to call for clarification of homework assignments.

- Parents, the biggest struggle is keeping on top of those dreaded long-range homework assignments (eg, reports, projects). This is something you will need to be vigilant about. Ask for a copy of the project requirements. Post the list at home and go over it together with your child. Write the due date on a master calendar. Then plan how to break down the project into manageable parts, scheduling steps along the way. Get started AT ONCE with going to the library, gathering resources, beginning the reading, and so forth.

Modified from: Rief S. *The ADD/ADHD Checklist: A Practical Reference for Parents & Teachers.* 2nd ed. 2008. This material used by permission of Jossey-Bass, a Wiley Imprint.

SUMMER SCHOOLS AND CAMPS

Many families have found it useful to supplement home- and school-based behavioral training techniques with a specially designed summer school or camp program for children with ADHD and their parents. The best of these programs focus on improving learning and academic achievement—developing children's abilities to follow through with instructions, complete tasks that they commonly fail to finish, and comply with adults' requests. They also help children develop problem-solving skills, social skills, and the social awareness needed to get along better with other children. Parents, meanwhile, are taught how to develop, reinforce, and maintain these positive changes. Summer programs also provide an excellent environment in which to carefully monitor and adjust doses of stimulant medication. However, these programs are typically expensive and the generalization and maintenance of benefits into the regular school setting may be limited.

A list of summer programs can be found on the Web site of the Center for Children and Families (http://ccf.buffalo.edu/stp.php). If no program exists in your area, the information on this site may help you advocate for one.

Medication Management

In addition to implementing behavioral training techniques that can help your child function successfully at school, your child's teacher is an essential resource in successfully managing medication issues—providing information that can help your child's treatment team decide whether to initiate medication, adjust the dosage, and so on. Your child's pediatrician should be in close contact with your child's teacher, calling him before each follow-up visit or reviewing the teacher's current written narrative or rating scales that reflect your child's academic, behavioral, and social functioning at school. Teachers need to be aware of what medications can and cannot be expected to do, as well as the possible adverse effects of any given medication. Your child's pediatrician may be able to provide his teacher with handouts explaining approaches to medication management as well as positive effects and side effects. As a parent, you can play a key case management role by encouraging this communication between your child's teacher and physician to make sure that they each get the information they need.

In most states, medications must be administered to students by a licensed medical provider, most often the school nurse—particularly because stimulant medications are legally considered controlled substances (see Chapter 4). Because many of the stimulant medications have "street value," it is usually not appropriate (or legal) for your child or adolescent to take them to school or to self-administer them, even if a particular school may be lenient in its policies. If medications are to be taken during the school day, make sure that you have filled out the appropriate consent forms for medication administration and that school personnel are informed immediately about any changes in dose or in the timing of doses. Keep in mind that several longer-acting medications are available and eliminate the need to take medications during the school day (see Chapter 4), allowing your child to avoid the problems of embarrassment and compliance issues associated with the administration of medication at school.

A Personal Coach/Trainer

If parents and teachers can be said to share one goal regarding children with ADHD, it is to help them learn to manage their own behavior and academic life so that they can enjoy an independent, happy adulthood. At first, most children with ADHD require a great deal of external monitoring because they are unable to provide it themselves. Gradually, with support and encouragement, they will begin to internalize this role. The concept of "coaching" has been developed over the past several years. The technique involves identifying a single person to serve as the child's daily monitor—briefly chatting with her each day, asking her what her most important tasks are for that day and how she plans to accomplish them, and praising her for working toward her goals. While parents have such conversations with their children as a matter of routine, a nonparent—a school employee, neighbor, friend's parent, responsible classmate, or even a hired college student or retired person— can sometimes have a greater impact simply because of their outsider status. The daily conversation between your child and her coach is brief and can take place by telephone. It might take place in the morning before the school day begins, in the evening before the child starts her homework, or at any other time that the child feels is most appropriate. Its effectiveness seems to spring from its combination of practical assistance with emotional support as well as the consistency and reliability of its presence in the child's life. While this brief, daily form of coaching does not replace the role of a parent, psychologist, pediatrician, or medication, it may make a substantive difference in a child's functioning at school. It can also take some of the tension out of day-to-day parent-child interactions when a more neutral party is helping to facilitate charged issues like homework flow. When meeting with your child's teacher, consider ask-ing him to recommend someone at school—a counselor, office clerk, or even a responsible student—who might be willing to act as coach for your child.

Support at Home

There is no denying that children with ADHD can make teaching, learning, and even play-ing more difficult at times. There is also no question that children with ADHD often have a special type of intensity, energy, and enthusiasm that can enhance everyone's daily experi-ence. As you support your child through her academic career, make a point of focusing on these positive qualities, and asking others to do so as well. Your child has much to contribute to her classroom and her school. Do what you can to help improve her chance for success in this challenging but potentially rewarding environment.

By the time they enter college, many students with ADHD have grown accustomed to seek-ing outside support, when necessary, such as special tutoring, coaching, altered testing con-ditions, or study environments, and tailoring their medication schedule to the demands of each semester's academic schedule. As these students demonstrate, the presence of ADHD does not spell the end of academic success, but will likely require careful planning in a well-informed and positive way.

Q & A

Q: *My six-year-old was recently diagnosed with hyperactive-impulsive–type ADHD. He had a great deal of difficulty with behavioral issues in kindergarten, and now his first-grade teacher has suggested that he might benefit from being held back a year before starting second grade. My son doesn't seem to be experiencing any academic problems so far. Is it a good idea to hold him back to allow him to learn to deal with behavioral issues?*

A: Parents of young children with ADHD—particularly kindergartners and first-graders—are frequently advised to allow their child to be held back a year to "catch up" on social skills or "grow out of" unsatisfactory behaviors. However, research does not support the notion that most children with ADHD will advance significantly in these areas as a result of being held back. In fact, repeating a grade can sometimes worsen behavior as boredom increases, prevent a child from receiving necessary special services because his performance resembles that of his younger classmates, and lead to self-esteem issues. For these reasons, most experts recommend advancing the child to the next grade while providing him with the support services he needs. These services might include behavior modification techniques, tutoring services, social-skills training within the school setting, or placement in a smaller classroom. Kindergartners may also benefit from moving into a kindergarten–first-grade transitional program combining kindergarten and first grade.

Q: *If it is determined that my child is eligible for Section 504 coverage, will she be automatically eligible for IDEA services as well?*

A: No. The 2 programs differ in their eligibility requirements and in their assessment and implementation processes. Your best plan would be to determine as best you can ahead of time which program is best suited to your child and request an evaluation under that program first. In general, a child with ADHD who requires special education services who has a coexisting disability or experiences serious and frequent behavior problems at school is best suited for IDEA coverage. A child whose needs are less severe may find suitable coverage under the less stringent and more inclusive requirements of Section 504.

Q: *Does my child have to be failing to qualify for special education services?*

A: No. Failing grades are a red flag for seeking extra help or special education services, but they are not a prerequisite for obtaining special services. The RTI services discussed in this chapter may be a road to securing valuable education services that may derail failure before it occurs.

Chapter 8

Advocating for Your Child and Others

An advocate can be broadly defined as "someone who speaks up to make things better." Advocates can speak up for themselves or others. You advocate each time you speak to teachers, care providers, physicians, nurses, social workers, or others. You are, in fact, the most important advocate for your child. When you combine your commitment to your child with effective advocacy skills, your child can become as independent and productive as possible.

Learning the skills needed to be an effective advocate can empower you as you help your child navigate life. As you advocate for your child to receive services and supports, remember that you are the expert on your child. Professionals have knowledge and expertise in specific areas, but your experience and long-term connection with your child is invaluable. Professionals will pass in and out of your child's life, but you will always be the parent. Your knowledge can be used to improve your child's life and even the lives of other families and children.

Advocating for your own child with attention-deficit/hyperactivity disorder (ADHD) can be the first step in learning how to advocate for many children. As an advocate, you can work to change "systems" as well as issues that affect your child. Every day, families of children with ADHD are affected by a variety of systems and how they operate: the school system, the health care system, government, or others. Most of the time these systems are helpful, but sometimes they may not adequately meet the needs of your child and other children. You may see the need to advocate for a system to change.

This chapter outlines how to be an effective advocate for your child and also provides information on systems advocacy. In the following pages you will learn about

- The 6 skills of an effective advocate
- Advocacy at school and with the health care system
- Advocacy for systems change

Six Skills of an Effective Advocate

Supporter, backer, believer, promoter—you are all of these when you advocate for your child. By using the 6 advocacy skills, you can become even more effective at promoting the interests of your child.

1. Understand Your Child's Disability

Understand all you can about your child's specific ADHD diagnosis. The knowledge you gather will allow you to ask educated, informed questions of your child's teachers and pediatricians. Also, as well as reading this book, you may consider joining support groups or specific organizations focused on ADHD, such as Children and Adults with Attention-Deficit/Hyperactivity Disorder (CHADD). Becoming acquainted with other adults who have ADHD can also be helpful. Their past experiences and current lives can provide you with "possible futures" for your child. The more you understand your child's specific diagnoses, the more you will be able to know if the services provided are appropriate to meet the needs of your child. The knowledge you gather will also allow you to ask educated, informed questions.

2. Know the Key Players

In order to influence someone to make a change you think is necessary for your child, you need to know the appropriate decision-maker. Who has the authority to make decisions that could lead to a change? Is it the Individualized Education Program (IEP) or social service case manager, a school administrator, a patient representative, or a city council member? If one person can't or won't help you, ask to speak to a person with more authority. To find the key players, ask for contact information; check the Internet, library, or phone book; and ask staff at your local parent advocacy or resource center for ideas.

3. Know Your Rights and Responsibilities

Knowing who is in charge is not enough. You also need to know the "rules" and participate from a position of knowledge as much as possible. Each agency, service provider, or school has guidelines for how it works. Each one has certain procedures, forms, policies, and sometimes laws and regulations that you will need to understand. Ask where you can find these in writing if available, and see what you can learn by reading the agency's or service's Web site. Because there is a direct link between how an agency or service is funded and what your specific rights and responsibilities are, it's also important to find the funding source. If the service is funded by the public, it is required to follow certain laws, not just policies. Publicly funded systems are supported by taxes and include public schools and all levels of government.

4. *Become Well Organized*

Most agencies and services require documents, data, and other records. It's important to organize the information and documents that you have and to be prepared by using the following tips:

- Separate your records by service or agency.
- Keep written correspondences, including printed e-mails, from school, county services, medical professionals, or any other system.
- Keep a list of names and contact numbers for each system you deal with.
- When you attend a meeting, bring the pertinent records from your file or folder.
- Keep records in order by date so you can easily find what you need.

It is always best to have as many things in writing as possible. This includes copies of any letters or e-mails you send yourself. People who have experience with advocacy have a saying: "If it's not in writing, it doesn't exist." If someone tells you something on the phone or in a hallway conversation that you feel is important, try to document it in writing. To do so, you might write a letter or e-mail saying, "Thank you for talking to me today. I think what you said was ＿＿ and that you will ＿＿. Unless I hear from you in writing by next week, I will assume you understood the conversation the same as I did." It is also helpful to keep a phone log and meeting notebook. Include the date, name of the person you talked with, a summary of what was said or decided, and brief notes of the issues that were discussed. If there were any specific things that you or the other person agreed to do, highlight them in your log so you can check on progress later.

If organization is not one of your strengths, you may wish to ask a family member or friend to help you organize these records.

5. *Use Clear and Effective Communication*

The way you talk to others has a direct relationship to how they interact with you and perhaps what services your child will receive. That's why it's important to make sure that your communication style is helping, and not hindering, your efforts. If you have a habit of expressing anger, for example, others will likely only remember that you were angry, not that you had good points or valid requests, and your child may not receive the help you were hoping for.

How would you define your communication attitude?

- Are you passive? (The professionals know more than I do; they won't listen so there is no need to speak up; I feel powerless and controlled by others.)

- Are you aggressive? (I know more than anyone else; I will make others fear me so I can achieve my goal; I don't care if I violate the rights of others.)

- Are you assertive? (I will share what I know; I will express my child's needs clearly; I will listen as others share what they know; I will feel heard.)

Strive to become an assertive communicator. To do that, you must first keep your eyes on the prize, which is effective service for your child. The focus should always be on your child and what your child needs, not what you need. Second, listen and ask questions. Listening gives you information that you will need. Whether you agree or not, try to understand what others are saying as you listen. To make sure you understand what the other person is saying, you might ask: "I think I heard you say _____. Is that correct?" Or, "Tell me more so I'm sure I understand your view." Asking questions is also important. If someone says "your child is disruptive," ask detailed questions about what they mean. What specifically does she do to be disruptive? When, and how often? Who or what does she disrupt? Knowing the answers to these questions will help determine a solution to the problem.

Effective communicators and advocates are as clear and direct as possible. They also turn negatives into positives. This technique allows you to take a negative comment made about your child and turn it into a positive. For example, "He's always fighting" could mean "It looks like my child needs to learn social skills."

At the end of a conversation it's important to summarize what you and others have said. Ask if you've misinterpreted or misunderstood anything, and ask to be corrected if you have. Ask if someone is writing down what was discussed and request a copy. Remember that good communicators focus on a goal, show respect and expect it from others, ask questions, rephrase what is said for clarification, and say thank you.

Communicating at a Meeting

You can problem-solve with professionals to find solutions using the following steps:

- Describe the problem clearly.
- Encourage input from all members of the team.
- Brainstorm without evaluating the ideas.
- Choose a solution by consensus.
- Develop a plan. Define who is responsible for an action and when it will be done.
- Put that plan in writing.
- Make sure that each item of the plan is clear and measurable so that you can track future progress.
- Create a timeline and criteria to evaluate success.
- Follow up to make sure the plan is implemented.

Written Communication

Clear written communication is also an important tool of effective advocates. Letters or e-mails may be sent for reasons, such as making a request, asking for clarification, clarifying what you said, asking for a decision, saying thank you, or documenting a verbal discussion. Use the following checklist when you write a letter or e-mail, and remember to keep a copy for yourself. Letters should

- Be sent to a person who can make a change
- Be dated and signed
- Focus on 1 or 2 issues
- Be no longer than 1 page
- Set a deadline if a reply is requested
- Give your contact information

6. *Know How to Resolve Disagreements*

As a parent, you may agree or disagree with the decisions made by an agency or service provider. Because of this, it's important to know how disagreements are settled within a specific organization. Each agency or service provider has formal or informal guidelines on how it works; each one has procedures, forms, policies, and sometimes laws and regulations. Ask if a given agency has a dispute resolution procedure and where you can find it in writing.

There are many ways to resolve disagreements. It's usually best to use informal means if possible. Start your efforts at the level closest to the problem. Talk to people, such as the teacher, case manager, or service provider, about your differences and be clear about why you do not agree. This often is the easiest way to solve a problem. Often, a compromise or "trial solution" can be worked out. Sometimes more formal means are necessary to clear up disagreements. Among the options may be

- **Mediation:** Agencies and service providers sometimes provide mediation. The parties who disagree meet with a neutral mediator and the mediator guides the discussion so that all sides and options can be heard.
- **Filing complaints:** Some agencies and service providers have a formal means of filing a grievance or complaint.
- **Filing appeals:** Some agencies and service providers have a written process for filing an appeal of a decision made by the agency or provider. All government agencies must have an appeals process. In addition, insurance companies also have appeals processes if a claim or procedure is denied.

At times, you may need to be "the squeaky wheel." Those who are persistent often receive the services their child or family needs.

Personal Advocacy at School

Advocating for your child at school usually involves attending meetings. Effective advocates prepare for these meetings, effectively communicate during the meetings, and try to end the meeting on a positive note.

Preparing for Meetings, Conferences, and Conversations

To be prepared, read your child's current evaluation report, IEP, and IEP goal progress reports. Think about what the issues are, and be ready to state them clearly. Consider ideas for a solution, and find specific facts to support your position. You will also want to make a list of your priorities and concerns before a meeting and be sure that they are listed on the meeting's agenda. Keep in mind that you may need to narrow your list since you may not be able to cover several issues at one meeting. You may wish to share your priority list with your child's case manager. To properly prepare, you can also write a list of questions and concerns, keeping in mind who will be at a meeting and what their roles will be. Make sure you know the purpose(s) of the meeting, and consider inviting someone to go with you to a meeting to help you remember the details of the discussion accurately. It's wise to inform the case manager if you do invite someone. You may also consider role-playing prior to a meeting—practicing what you intend to say in front of a friend, colleague, or relative who can also ask you some challenging questions that you might encounter. By using this technique, you can think out and articulate your answers before having to state them in public. Prepare your role-playing approach by anticipating what will be discussed at the IEP meeting or school conference.

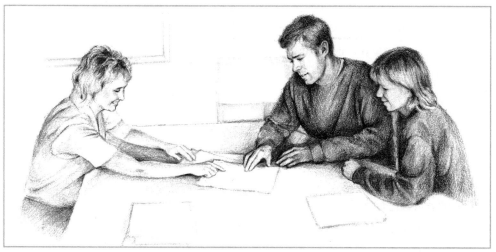

When you attend a meeting, be sure to bring important records from your file. To help prepare, make a list of questions in advance of the meeting.

Beginning a Meeting

To set the stage for an effective meeting

- Arrive early enough to sit where you will feel most comfortable and effective. Consider the advisability of bringing your child to the meeting. If your child does not attend, bring a picture and place it on the table.
- Establish rapport. Tell a short, interesting story about your child. Handshakes, small talk, and smiles can open a meeting on a positive note.
- Seek common ground. Start with things that team members agree on.
- Make sure there is an agenda and that it includes your items.
- Find out how much time has been scheduled for this meeting. Is it enough?

During the Meeting

- Identify and focus on your goal. Hold yourself accountable.
- Show respect, expect it from others, and remain calm.
- Be specific and clear. Instead of "He follows directions at home," you may want to say, "At home he follows directions better when I give him two-step directions with one reminder."
- Acknowledge that you understand that teachers have multiple and complex roles.
- Ask questions if unfamiliar terms are used or unfamiliar district policies are mentioned.
- Take notes on what you hear or invite a friend to do this for you.
- Don't interrupt. Allow the speaker to finish; don't assume you know what the speaker will say.
- Don't "argue mentally." You may miss some data or the real message while thinking of what you will say next.
- Use praise and say thanks whenever possible.
- Rephrase what you hear to ensure you understood correctly.

Ending a Meeting

End a meeting by summarizing its results. By doing this, you can make sure you understood correctly and can clarify who will do what by when. End on a positive note whenever possible. Even if you've disagreed, you may be able to say, "I think we understand each other's perspectives more clearly now."

Other Tips for Effective School Meetings

Use "This will..." instead of "I think...." Example: "Seating Jimmy in the front row and away from the window will help him focus on his work." versus "I think Jimmy needs to sit somewhere else." The first statement offers a concrete reason to consider your suggestion while the second statement is an opinion.

Use "You could..." rather than "You should...." Examples: "Instead of sending Tara to the office, you could call the social worker." versus "You should never send Tara to the office." "Jon's progress in learning to read seems very slow. Could we look at other methods?" versus "You should use a different method for teaching reading." The first statements suggest an option that's open to discussion and flexibility. The second statements imply that you are ordering someone to do something.

Use "I" Statements

Here are some examples: "I would like to talk about what my daughter is learning." "I feel like I'm not being heard." "I didn't understand that. I'd like to stop and go back."

Leave Out the Word "You"

Using the word "you" in a sentence can cause other people to feel defensive. Defensive people don't listen because they are busy thinking of ways to defend themselves. This accomplishes nothing positive for the child. Example: "You are not helping my daughter." versus "My daughter is not getting the help she needs."

Phrases that may improve communication include

- "Tell me more about...."
- "That term (or acronym) is unfamiliar to me. Would you please define it?"
- "Please explain...."
- "Would you please rephrase that so I can understand?"
- "How will I know this plan is working?"
- "What will the school propose to do about...?"
- "What do you suggest we do about...?"
- "I think I heard you say.... Is that correct?"

- "How was that progress you mentioned measured?"
- "That is interesting. Tell me more so I'm sure I understand your view."
- "How long will we need to use this intervention to determine if it is successful?"

Personal Advocacy Within the Health Care System

The first step in advocating for your child in the health care system is making sure you have a positive relationship with a compassionate and qualified physician. Consider whether your child's doctor meets the following basic expectations: Does the doctor show respect for you and your child, show a willingness to listen patiently, take your concerns seriously, have courteous office staff, and support your goals for your child? Throughout your relationship with the doctor, you should think about whether these basic expectations are being met. As a parent, you must also do your part to ensure a good relationship and good communication with your child's physician. As you work with your child's physician, keep the following things in mind:

- Remain realistic about what you can expect of your child's physician. Remember that one doctor cannot solve all of the problems or answer all of your questions.
- Doctors are human and, like you, may occasionally be frustrated by gaps in knowledge about ADHD or the lack of answers to questions. Let your child's doctor know that you appreciate the extra time given to you and your child and the extra work involved in caring for your child.
- Keeping in mind the medical home model, you are part of the health care team, participating in decision-making about your child's care. This means that you have responsibilities for communicating effectively with your child's physician, keeping records, and following up.

Advocating for good health care and communicating well with your child's doctor is easier if you are prepared and organized.

Before an Appointment

- Keep a journal. Write down your observations of behavior, reactions to medications, sleep patterns, eating habits, or anything else that your physician may need to know.

- Keep medical records. You have the right to copies of your child's medical records. Keep your own records of tests and procedures, and their results. You can do this by dividing a 3-ring binder into relevant sections, such as current care plan, providers' names, health history, current and past medications, addresses and phone numbers, bills, referrals, insurance information, and appointment logs. Premade medical record systems are also available, as well as online medical organizers.
- Write out questions. Do not hesitate to ask questions and do not be embarrassed to ask for clarification when you don't understand something the doctor says.
- Prepare your child. Tell your child what to expect, who you will be seeing and why, and what tests may be done. Take comfort items along on the appointment.

During the Appointment

Make an effort to understand the doctor—listen and take notes. Ask the doctor to explain the treatment plan and put it in writing, repeat the care plan back to the doctor as you understand it, and ask questions. If the doctor does not have the time to answer all of your questions or needs time to look into the matter, give the doctor a written list of questions and ask that he or she call you to continue the discussion. Ask the doctor to set a time frame.

After the Appointment

Ask for a second opinion from another doctor if you feel it is needed. If you are uncertain or uncomfortable about a diagnosis or treatment, follow your instincts about your child and talk more with the physician about your concern. You may feel it's necessary to change doctors. Some reasons for selecting another medical professional are if the doctor is not responsive to your concerns, is not listening to you and your child, is not communicating with specialists, or is not helping you coordinate your child's care.

Insurance Coverage and Appealing Health Plan Decisions

To be an effective advocate for your child's needs within the guidelines of your health plan, you will need to understand the plan. Carefully read your health plan policy, certificate of coverage, health benefits handbook, or other documents that explain your policy's benefits as well as its coverage limits. As you review the plan, note which services are and are not covered, and read the "definitions" section so you understand unfamiliar terms. If you have coverage questions, call the health plan's customer service line, which can be found on the back of your member card and in your benefit handbook. You may want to ask

- Do I need a referral from my child's primary care physician to see a specialist?
- Must I use a preferred list of network providers?
- What if I want to see someone outside that network?
- Is there an annual deductible?
- Are there limits on the number of visits?
- Does the plan exclude certain diagnoses or preexisting conditions?
- Is there a lifetime dollar limit?
- What is my prescription coverage?

As with other areas of advocacy, it's important to keep good records. Record the date, time, and name of the person you spoke with on any calls to or from your health plan. Take notes on the conversation and the information you were given. Verify that the information provided over the phone agrees with your policy.

Developing a strong relationship with your child's pediatrician is also beneficial when dealing with insurance coverage and any appeals process. Contact your child's primary physician if you need help with referrals or appeals, and always involve your child's pediatrician in the coordination of care. This will ensure smooth delivery of services and good communication among all providers. Be sure that requests, referrals, or orders for services come from a physician. Requests from a therapist or licensed psychologist may not be accepted by health plans.

Denial of Insurance Claims

If coverage for services for your child is denied, first make sure the denial is legitimate. Compare the reason stated in the denial letter to your certificate of coverage. You should also make certain that any denials are in writing, not in person or over the phone.

If you've determined that the denial matches the rules set out in your health care plan, consider the reason for the denial. If services are denied because they're not covered under your plan, explore whether the plan is clear about its exclusions and whether any exceptions are allowed. If services are denied because they're not considered medically necessary, consider filing an appeal based on factual reasons why the services are necessary for your child. Your child's pediatrician or primary care provider can help you with this information.

Appealing Health Plan Decisions

If you choose to appeal a decision of your health plan, you will need to understand the appeal process and give the health plan as much information as possible to support your claim. All health plans are required by law to have an appeal process. You will find information about your plan's appeal process by reading your policy or certificate of coverage or by contacting your health plan and asking for a written copy of the appeal process. Your plan will send you a letter that explains why your request has been denied. Read the reasons carefully so you can prepare a strong appeal.

In most cases, in order to start the appeal process you must submit the appeal in writing. Use these guidelines to organize your letter.

- **Purpose:** State your purpose for writing.
- **Diagnosis:** Explain your child's diagnosis and how it affects your child.
- **Reasons:** Give specific reasons why your child needs the service.
- **Documentation:** Mention the supporting documentation you are including.
- **Action:** Close by requesting a written reply.

Strengthen your appeal by including written support from your child's medical providers explaining why your child needs the services requested. Ask for letters of support from one or more doctors familiar with your child's case. It is also helpful to create a paper trail by organizing your policy, copies of denial letters, copies of any correspondence with your health plan, detailed notes of conversations (date and time of call, name of person you spoke with, what was discussed), and copies of any correspondence between your physician and the health plan concerning your problem. Finally, send copies of all correspondence with your plan to all interested persons. For example, you may send copies to your physician and anyone else you have contacted regarding your situation. Indicate that you have sent copies by noting each name at the bottom of the letter under "cc."

Strengthening your advocacy skills will benefit your child now and in the future and will help you secure needed supports and services for your child. Some parents take advocacy a step further and use their personal stories, skills, and knowledge to push for changes that will improve the lives of other children with ADHD.

Systems Advocacy

Many parents begin the journey from personal advocacy toward systems advocacy after they are faced with payment limitations and regulations that limit services and supports for their child. Because they have the "lived experience" of parenting a child with ADHD, they know what works and what doesn't work in a system. They see a need to change a "system," specifically the policies, laws, or rules that determine how services will be provided to families of children with disabilities. Unhappy with the way the health care system or public school system has responded to their needs, these parents seek new ways to address their concerns. They begin working with others, including national support groups and advocacy organizations, to make large-scale improvements. As a systems change advocate, you too can speak up to improve services for all children with ADHD and their families. You can learn to advocate for meaningful changes that may affect thousands of children in your community, state, or throughout the country.

Many systems impact the families of children with disabilities. Each system has a certain way of operating, whether it's a school; a faith-based organization; a hospital; a health insurance company; a community center; or the city, county, state, and federal government. To change how a system operates, parents need to understand how it works. This is not always easy, especially within the public policy arena. Working for change within the American intergovernmental system of federalism (national, state, and local governments) and American constitutional separation of governmental powers (legislative, executive, and judicial branches) can be daunting. That's why most advocates of systems change turn to allies— those in a similar position who are dealing with the same issue, such as the way the health care system and the public school system treats disability.

Despite the challenges, many individuals have stepped forward, joined together, and made changes at the system level that now provide basic educational and civil rights for people with disabilities. If you choose to follow in their footsteps and work for systems change, follow these first important steps.

- **Link with others and build relationships.** Who in your school, family, neighborhood, or faith community is facing similar limitations and frustrations? Seek them out. It's particularly effective to connect with families who are already involved in health, education, and disability advocacy—they can teach you.

- **Connect to organizations doing public policy work.** The American Pluralistic Society is a dynamic scene of support groups, many of which focus on particular disabilities and work to change public policy for the benefit of children and adults with disabilities. Many of these groups have public policy advocacy positions and are a natural place to go for support and to become involved. In the area of ADHD, CHADD is one such group (www.chadd.org). There are also more than 100 parent training and information centers and community parent resource centers throughout the United States that provide information and support for families of children with disabilities, as well as advocacy support. PACER Center (Parent Advocacy Coalition for Educational Rights) is the Technical Assistance Alliance for Parent Centers (http://www.taalliance.org /) and a source of information for parents on advocacy. To find a parent center in your state, visit PACER.org and click on National Parent Centers.

- **Learn public policy facts.** Public policy is a daunting and complex arena. The support groups identified above, particularly those physically located in the nation's capital and the state government capitals, are a wealth of factual information. Even if you disagree with the philosophy and policy agenda of a support group, you can learn much by reading the facts posted on its Web site. In addition to support and family advocacy groups, professional and trade associations are a good source of information. Again, you may not always agree with your school principal, your school psychologist, and your health insurance plan, but their professional and trade associations have much information.

Legislative Advocacy

Laws in America are written by legislative bodies. To advocate for a change in the law, you must work with the people in those bodies, which include the US Congress, state legislatures, county councils, city councils, and school boards. Most legislative bodies have their own Web sites, and you can use them to research the existing laws governing health care, public education, and disability. The support and advocacy groups previously discussed also have information on legislation and legislative bodies.

To advocate for change, you will need to convey your message to the appropriate legislators. Because America's legislative members represent geographic areas, legislators respond best to their constituents (the voters from that area). Constituents carry influence. Your first task is to determine which legislators represent your area.

Once you know who your legislators are, tell them your personal story. Legislators need to know how a particular public program is affecting or limiting the welfare and needs of your family. If possible, relate your personal story to the personal stories of others and work in coalitions and partnerships. When advocating, don't forget to ask yourself: Who is it I want to persuade? What seems important to them? How can my personal story relate to that person I want to persuade? Educating legislative members about health, education, and disability by telling your personal story is important.

Dos and don'ts for dealing with your legislators include

Do

- Be concise and clear. Legislators are busy and hear from many people. Can you tell your story in 5 minutes?
- Stick to one issue. What is the one take-away message they should remember?
- Provide a handout to help deliver the message. The "leave behind" document is important. Try to limit the length to no more than one sheet (front and back of one sheet).
- Send them a thank-you letter and stay in contact with their office.
- Join coalitions. Many other people will be contacting their legislators, frequently on the same issue. Being part of an organization and having your organization working in coalitions builds numbers and increases information. Consistency of message is more likely to garner a legislator's support. Mention to legislators the other organizations, coalitions, and constituents that you are working with. Legislators want to know that you are not alone—that other constituents are concerned with the same issues (and hopefully have the same advocacy positions).

Don't

- Mix causes and messages. Don't share your views on a wide variety of issues and concerns.
- Threaten, offend, preach, or write off anyone. You will meet legislators and their staff who aren't supportive or interested. State your case and be polite. Try to be a good listener regarding what they care about and why.
- Be late for appointments. This may be a particular challenge for many persons with ADHD.
- Guess about answers. If you don't know something when they ask, say you don't know and will get back to them.

Advocating in the Health Care System

America's health care system, which is one-sixth of the US economy, is extremely complex. Trying to figure out who pays can be difficult. Many Americans are enrolled in more than one health care program. Each program has its own legal and regulatory requirements and limitations. The largest and most important health care payment programs and the number of Americans they insure are

- Employer-paid health insurance: 158 million Americans; 53% of the US population
- Federal employee health benefits program: 8 million federal employees, retirees, former employees, and their families; 2.7% of the US population
- Other private insurance (non-employer paid): 15 million Americans; 5% of the US population
- Medicare: 42 million Americans; 14% of the US population
- Medicaid: 39 million Americans; 13% of the US population
- State Children's Health Insurance Program (SCHIP): 7.4 million Americans; 2.5% of the US population
- Veterans Administration's Health Care System: 7.84 million; 2.6% of the US population

Additionally, there are specialized health care delivery programs such as Tri-Care (formerly known as CHAMPUS) for active duty personnel and their families, federally qualified health centers for medically underserved populations, and state mental health authorities serving the most severely disabled by mental illness and children with mental health challenges.

It is easier to influence public sector health programs, which are provided by the government, than private sector health programs, which are private insurance plans paid by employers.

Public programs are authorized by federal and state law and sometimes complemented by county governments. Government agencies issue regulations governing these programs. Typically, there is a public comment period on proposed regulations, which allows advocates to share their viewpoints. Increasingly, contracts between government agencies and health plans are available by the public, which helps advocates be informed. Most states have consumer protections and consumer rights laws and regulations, including internal and external appeals procedures that can allow advocates to work for change. A fundamental barrier to receiving needed health services is the definition of "medical necessity." The definition of "medical necessity" is frequently held "confidential" to the health plan decision-makers, but can be challenged by treating professionals on behalf of consumers and their families. Another quasi-public barrier is medication formularies. These can be challenged by treating professionals on behalf of their consumers and their families.

In the private sector, one way you may advocate for change is through state law. Many states have laws providing consumer grievance procedures against health plans in the private sector.

Probably the best single source of consumer-oriented health rights information is the National Health Law Program (www.healthlaw.org). A very helpful consumer guide is the National Alliance on Mental Illness (www.nami.org) *Legal Protections and Advocacy Strategies for People with Severe Mental Illnesses in Managed Care Systems* (available at http://www.nami.org/Content/ContentGroups/Legal/ManagedCare.pdf).

A major systems advocacy objective of the American Academy of Pediatrics (AAP), actively supported by CHADD, is adoption of the medical home. A medical home is a single medical practice taking ownership and responsibility to coordinate interventions for children with special needs. The focus is on the whole child, youth, and family with coordinated care/services/supports. The federal Maternal and Child Health Bureau currently funds the AAP-supported medical home models throughout the country, and the pending national health care reform legislation would greatly expand these models.

A Success Story

Systems advocacy can be successful if individual advocates join with advocacy groups and coalitions and patiently continue their efforts with a united front. A major change in health care law was recently accomplished following a 2-decade effort by the entire national mental health movement, joined through coalition in the more recent years by the national substance abuse community. Their advocacy efforts succeeded on October 3, 2008, when President George W. Bush signed the Paul Wellstone and Pete Domenici Mental Health Parity and Addiction Equity Act into law. (On February 2, 2010, the US Departments of Health and Human Services, Labor, and Treasury issued interim final regulations implementing the act. Details are available at www.chadd.org. Click on the Influencing Policy link from the home page and then Mental Health Parity.)

The Mental Health Parity Act requires health insurance companies to treat mental illnesses and disorders on an equal basis with physical illnesses and disorders, when polices cover both. Until 2010 most health insurance plans in America treated mental disorders in a discriminatory fashion compared with physical disorders. For example, the typical health insurance plan in America authorizes unlimited hospitalization for physical disorders while limiting hospitalization for mental health disorders to 30 days per calendar year; it authorizes a broad array of outpatient services for physical insurance but limits outpatient mental health services, particularly relevant to children and adolescents diagnosed with ADHD, to 20 visits each year; and it requires a 20% copayment for health services, while frequently requiring mental health copayments of 50%. All of these forms of discrimination will end in large- and medium-sized health plans.

This new law, which is the product of many national organizations working in coalition over many years with the same public policy objective, proves that people can change systems and laws if they unite and persevere in their efforts.

Advocacy Makes a Difference

You can be an advocate for systems change while continuing to personally advocate for your family member. Whether you are learning how to be a better advocate for your child or delving into systems advocacy, know that advocacy of all types is an art—the art of persuasion. Being knowledgeable, honest, polite, and persistent are important tools of this art. As demonstrated with the 2-decade effort to pass mental health parity legislation, patience is required for systems change, and working with others for common objectives is almost always necessary. Remember, you are not alone in your desire to make positive changes for your child and others. There are many family-oriented organizations, working in concert with professional organizations, to improve the lives of persons with disabilities, including those with ADHD and related disorders. The Washington office of the AAP, for example, is a model of knowledge, partnership with families, and effectiveness.

For some, public policy advocacy can be a frustrating experience, but many find it to be an exciting, dynamic activity. When you engage in systems advocacy, you'll find persons who share your interest in promoting the public welfare and helping other families overcome their challenges. Children with disabilities receive services today based on the past advocacy work of parents like you and professionals. You can add your important voice to improve the services for children and families today and tomorrow.

Chapter 9

When It Is Not Just ADHD: Identifying Coexisting Conditions

Attention-deficit/hyperactivity disorder (ADHD) often occurs with coexisting conditions. Fifty percent to 60% of children with ADHD have at least one coexisting condition. More than 10% of children with ADHD have 3 or more coexisting conditions. Disruptive behavior disorders (disorders involving behavior and conduct problems), anxiety and depressive disorders, learning disabilities, and language impairments are the most common.

Coexisting conditions may share many of the same symptoms or mimic the symptoms of ADHD. Coexisting conditions in young children with ADHD are particularly hard to identify correctly because children's behavior changes quickly and certain conditions only become diagnosable over time. What seemed at 4 years of age to be a developing mood disorder may turn out to be aspects of ADHD.

In addition to diagnosed disorders, many children with ADHD experience coexisting "problems"—functioning difficulties that are not formally defined as disabilities but that still require special attention. For example, up to 60% of children with ADHD experience some form of academic problem in school subjects (reading, math, social studies, etc), skills (such as handwriting), or productivity (completing assignments accurately and on time), and most of these children do not have learning disorders.

In many cases—as with learning disorders that impede school performance—a coexisting condition or problem may affect your child's functioning in ways that require changes in his education or treatment plan. Sometimes, as can be the case with major depressive disorder (MDD), the symptoms of the coexisting condition may be more problematic than those of the ADHD and must be treated first, even if the ADHD was the original cause of your child's referral for treatment. In addition, a child's environment may play an important role. The behavior of a child with ADHD may, at times, cause stress within the family or may reflect stress within the family, resulting in greater severity of the child's symptoms.

Some conditions, such as conduct disorder, which involves extreme defiance and flaunting of rules, carry increased risks for substance abuse, criminal behavior, or other difficulties later in life—risks that may be diminished or even avoided if the condition is identified early and treated. For all of these reasons, it is always necessary to consider whether any of these coexisting conditions are present when your child is being evaluated for ADHD, and a comprehensive evaluation and ongoing monitoring are needed to diagnose any additional conditions and problems that can accompany ADHD. Continued monitoring is vital throughout childhood and adolescence because some coexisting conditions may develop long after the original ADHD diagnosis and others may diminish over time. In this chapter you will find information on how best to recognize and treat the types of coexisting conditions that most commonly accompany ADHD, including

- **Disruptive behavior disorders,** including oppositional defiant disorder (ODD) and conduct disorder (CD)
- **Anxiety disorders,** such as generalized anxiety disorder, separation anxiety disorder, phobias, and post-traumatic stress disorders
- **Mood disorders,** including MDD, dysthymia, and bipolar disorder
- **Tics, Tourette disorder, and obsessive-compulsive disorder (OCD)**
- **Learning, motor skills, and communication disorders**
- **Intellectual disability (formerly called mental retardation)**
- **Autism spectrum disorders (ASDs), pervasive developmental disorders (PPDs),** such as autism and related disorders
- **Coexisting problems** that, while not reaching the severity required for a specific diagnosis, may still significantly stand in the way of your child's progress

There are other problems that might either look very similar to ADHD, or make the symptoms of ADHD stand out more. These include

- Sensory deficits, such as hearing or vision problems
- Sleep deprivation
- Bereavement
- Certain physical illnesses (eg, thyroid disease, hypoglycemia, hyperglycemia, side effects of medications, and endocrine tumors)

- Substance use or withdrawal from substances
- Exposure to adverse childhood experiences

When viewed all together, this list of disorders may seem daunting, and even frightening. Keep in mind, however, that although concurrent conditions occur in most children and adolescents with ADHD, no child has all of these conditions, and most are treatable. With early identification and a systematic evidence-based treatment program, you and your child may be able to avoid or minimize many of the effects of disorders that do appear. Furthermore, the strengths of your child and family are important factors in increasing the likelihood that he will function well, despite these conditions.

What Else Is Going On? Recognizing and Diagnosing Coexisting Disorders

Identifying a coexisting condition can be difficult because many behaviors suggestive of these conditions—such as sadness, anxiety, or frequent rule breaking—could also stem from ADHD-related difficulties, responses to conflict at home or at school, or just a normal part of the process of growing up. Your child may frequently seem defiant and uncooperative for many reasons. As with ADHD, there are no laboratory tests to determine whether his behavior is due to a coexisting condition. An accurate diagnosis may involve a combination of factors, including a review of your careful observations of your child's behavior, an interview with your child, regular discussions among all members of his treatment and education teams, a review of your family's medical history, and the use of other tests or standardized rating scales as appropriate. Even with these aids, categorizing your child's cluster of behaviors as ADHD alone, as ADHD plus a coexisting condition, or even as a separate condition without ADHD may require multiple perspectives and regular review. If your child has already been diagnosed with ADHD but has shown little or no response to systematic trials of medication and behavior therapy techniques, or you have increasingly observed symptoms of the specific disorders described later in this chapter, he may have one or more coexisting conditions or problems in addition to ADHD. If your child was very young when he was diagnosed with ADHD, it may even turn out that he has the other disorder and not ADHD. If you are beginning to question whether your child has a coexisting condition and is not just functioning poorly due to stresses or frustrations directly related to ADHD, ask yourself

- **How long has the troublesome behavior lasted?** Has oppositional behavior been going on for longer than about 6 months? Particularly in younger children, troublesome behavior can come and go quickly—but if your child's difficulties persist beyond half a year, he may need assessment for a coexisting condition. In the case of depression or anxiety symptoms, an even shorter observation period is recommended.
- **Is the behavior typical of her age group?** Troublesome behavior occurs in all children during various stages of development. Assessment may be necessary, however, if your child's problems develop or persist long past the age when others her age have outgrown such behavior.
- **How intense is the behavior?** All children test boundaries, act fearful, or are depressed now and then, but children with a diagnosable condition act in more prolonged and intense ways than others their age.
- **How much of a problem is it causing in his day-to-day functioning?** Is the behavior significantly interfering with your child's academic progress, social relationships, or other important aspects of daily life? If so, a coexisting condition may be the cause.
- **Do you see any developmental delays?** Particularly during your child's preschool and early school years, keep track of whether he reaches the standard developmental milestones listed on child development charts at or around the ages indicated. Your child's pediatrician will be checking on these during your well-child visits, and they are included in most child care books. Watch especially for any significant delays in language development, social skills, motor skills, or academic progress.
- **Do others in your child's family have ADHD or one or more of the conditions listed in this chapter?** Many coexisting conditions run in families. A child with ADHD and a close relative with conditions such as an anxiety disorder, depression, learning disorders, oppositional behavior, or a more serious conduct disorder has a greater chance of having ADHD and/or a coexisting condition himself.

If your answers to any of these questions have left you with doubts or even questions about your child's functioning, be sure to discuss your observations with your child's pediatrician, and any other professionals involved with your child's care. If the diagnosis of ADHD has been made, your doctor should evaluate your child for any coexisting conditions, including those that could require additional or alternative treatment. In some cases, like in a child with ADHD plus a serious mood or anxiety disorder, the pediatrician may refer your child to a subspecialist to help in the diagnosis and management of his condition. So if your child has OCD along with ADHD, for example, a cognitive-behavioral therapist may be best equipped to help him in this aspect of his care, while the pediatrician oversees treatment of the ADHD. If your child has a very serious condition—such as a debilitating depression—this may need immediate treatment, even before your pediatrician begins treatment for the ADHD.

Following are the types of behaviors that are likely to signal each type of coexisting disorder, and the changes in treatment that may be necessary to address the coexisting disorder along with ADHD. In some cases, treatment of the ADHD itself may actually resolve the coexisting condition.

Disruptive Behavior Disorders

Disruptive behavior disorders are among the easiest to identify of all coexisting conditions because they involve behaviors that are readily seen, such as temper tantrums, physical aggression like attacking other children, excessive argumentativeness, stealing, and other forms of defiance or resistance to authority. These disorders, which include ODD and CD, often first attract notice when they interfere with school performance or family and peer relationships, and frequently intensify over time.

Behaviors typical of disruptive behavior disorders can closely resemble ADHD—particularly where impulsivity and hyperactivity are involved—but ADHD, ODD, and CD are considered separate conditions that can occur independently. About one-third of all children with ADHD have coexisting ODD, and up to one-quarter have coexisting CD. Children with both conditions tend to have more difficult lives than those with ADHD alone because their defiant behavior leads to so many conflicts with adults and others with whom they interact. Early identification and treatment may, however, increase the chances that your child can learn to control these behaviors.

Oppositional Defiant Disorder

Many children with ADHD display oppositional behaviors at times. Oppositional defiant disorder is defined in the American Psychiatric Association's *Diagnostic and Statistical Manual of Mental Disorders, Fourth Edition, Text Revision (DSM-IV-TR)* as including persistent symptoms of "negativistic, defiant, disobedient, and hostile behaviors toward authority figures." A child with ODD may argue frequently with adults; lose his temper easily; refuse to follow rules; blame others for his own mistakes; deliberately annoy others; and otherwise behave in angry, resentful, and vindictive ways. He is likely to encounter frequent social conflicts and disciplinary situations at school. In many cases, particularly without early diagnosis and treatment, these symptoms worsen over time—sometimes becoming severe enough to eventually lead to a diagnosis of CD.

Conduct Disorder

Conduct disorder is a more extreme condition than ODD. Defined in the *DSM-IV-TR* as "a repetitive and persistent pattern of behavior in which the basic rights of others or major age-appropriate social rules are violated," CD may involve serious aggression toward people or the hurting of animals, deliberate destruction of property (vandalism), stealing, running away from home, skipping school, or otherwise trying to break some of the major rules of society without getting caught. Many children with CD were or could have been diagnosed with ODD at an earlier age—particularly those who were physically aggressive when they were younger. As the CD symptoms become evident, these children usually retain their ODD symptoms (argumentativeness, resistance, etc) as well. This cluster of behaviors, combined with the impulsiveness and hyperactivity of ADHD, sometimes causes these children to be viewed as delinquents, and they are likely to be suspended from school and have more police contact than children and adolescents with ADHD alone or ADHD with ODD.

Children with ADHD whose CD symptoms started at an early age also tend to fare more poorly in adulthood than those with ADHD alone or ADHD with ODD—particularly in the areas of delinquency, illegal behavior, and substance abuse. However, early and effective treatment can prevent later problems of delinquency, illegal behavior, and substance abuse.

Oppositional Defiant Disorder and Conduct Disorder: What to Look For

A child with ADHD and a coexisting disruptive behavior disorder is likely to be similar to children with ADHD alone in terms of intelligence, medical history, and neurologic development. He is probably no more impulsive than children with ADHD alone, although if he has CD, his teachers or other adults may misinterpret his aggressive behavior as ADHD-type impulsiveness. However, the behavior of children with ADHD does not typically involve this level of aggression. A child with ADHD and CD does have a greater chance of experiencing learning disabilities, such as reading disorders and verbal impairment. But what distinguishes children with ODD and CD most from children with ADHD alone is their defiant, resistant, even (in the case of CD) aggressive, cruel, or delinquent, behavior. Other indicators to look for include

- **Relatives with ADHD/ODD, ADHD/CD, depressive disorder, or anxiety disorder.** A child with family members with ADHD/ODD or ADHD/CD should be watched for ADHD/CD as well. Chances of developing CD are also greater if family members have experienced depressive, anxiety, or learning disorders.
- **Stress or conflict in the family.** Divorce, separation, substance abuse, parental criminal activity, or serious conflicts within the family are common among children with ADHD and coexisting ODD or CD.
- **Poor or no positive response to the behavior therapy techniques at home and at school.** If your child defies your instructions, violates time-out procedures, and otherwise refuses to cooperate with your use of appropriate behavior therapy techniques, and his aggressive behavior continues, he should be evaluated for coexisting ODD or CD.

Treatment

Children with ADHD and disruptive behavior disorders often benefit from special behavioral techniques that can be implemented at home and at school. These approaches typically include methods for teaching your child to become more aware of his own anger cues, and using these cues as signals to initiate various coping strategies ("Take five deep breaths and think about the three best choices for how to respond before lashing out at a teacher."), and for providing himself with positive reinforcement (telling himself, "Good job, you caught the signal and used your strategies!") for successful self-control. You and your child's teachers, meanwhile, can learn to better manage ODD- or CD-type behavior through negotiating, compromising, problem-solving with your child, anticipating and avoiding potentially explosive situations, and prioritizing goals so that less important problems are ignored until more pressing issues have been successfully addressed. These highly specific techniques can be taught by professional behavior therapists or other mental health professionals recommended by your child's pediatrician or school psychologist, or other professionals involved with your family.

If your child has been diagnosed with coexisting ODD or CD, and well-planned classroom behavioral techniques in his mainstream classroom have been ineffective, this may lead to a decision to place him in a special classroom at school that is set up for more intensive behavior management. However, schools are mandated to educate your child in a mainstream classroom if possible, and to regularly review your child's education plan and reassess the appropriateness of his placement. It is very advisable, if possible, to keep your child in an environment where appropriate behaviors are being modeled day by day, rather than a classroom where inappropriate behaviors are frequent.

There is growing evidence that the same stimulant medications that improve the core ADHD symptoms may also help with coexisting ODD and CD. Stimulants have been shown to help decrease verbal and physical aggression, negative peer interactions, stealing, and vandalism. Although stimulant medications do not teach children new skills, such as helping them identify and respond appropriately to others' social signals, they may decrease the aggression that stands in the way of forming relationships with others their age. For this reason, stimulants are usually the first choice in a medication treatment approach for children with ADHD and a coexisting disruptive behavior disorder.

The earlier that stimulants are introduced to treat coexisting ODD or CD, the better. A child with a disruptive behavior disorder whose aggressive behavior continues untreated may start to identify with others who experience discipline problems. By adolescence, he may resist treatment that could help him change his behavior and make him less popular among these friends. He will have grown accustomed to his defiant "self" and feel uncomfortable and "unreal" when stimulants help check his reckless, authority-flaunting style. By treating these behaviors in elementary school or even earlier, you may have a better chance of preventing your child from creating a negative self-identity.

If your child has been treated with 2 or more types of stimulants and his aggressive symptoms are the same or worse, his pediatrician may choose to reevaluate the situation and replace the stimulants with other medications. If stimulant medication alone led to some but not enough improvement, his pediatrician may continue to prescribe stimulants in combination with one of these other agents. Finding and learning behavioral management methods that work, however, is always a central approach for an overall treatment plan.

Anxiety Disorders

As with disruptive behavior disorders, there is a great deal of overlap between anxiety disorders and ADHD. About one-fourth of children with ADHD also have an anxiety disorder. Likewise, about one-fourth of children with anxiety disorders have ADHD. This includes all types of anxiety disorders—generalized anxiety disorder, OCD, separation anxiety, and phobia (including social anxiety). Younger children who are overanxious or with separation anxiety are especially likely to also have ADHD.

Anxiety disorders are often more difficult to recognize than disruptive behavior disorders because the former's symptoms are *internalized*—that is, they often exist within the mind of the child rather than in outward behavior, such as verbal outbursts or pushing others to be first in line. An anxious child may be experiencing guilt, fear, or even irritability and yet escape notice by a parent, teacher, or pediatrician. Only when his symptoms are expressed in actual behavior, such as sleeplessness, or refusal to attend school, will he attract the attention he needs. It is important to ask your child's pediatrician or psychologist to talk with your child directly if you suspect the presence of persistent anxiety in addition to his ADHD.

OPPOSITONAL DEFIANT AND CONDUCT PROBLEM MEASURES THAT PARENTS CAN TAKE

Promote daily positive messages to your child.

• Praise compliant behavior—"Catch them being good."

• Encourage praise and rewards for specific, agreed, desired (target) behaviors.

Focus on prevention in the following ways:

• When possible, reorganize your child's day to prevent trouble by avoiding situations in which the child cannot control himself or herself. Examples include asking a neighbor to look after your child while you go shopping, ensuring that activities are available for long car journeys, and arranging activities in separate rooms for siblings who are prone to fight.

• Monitor the whereabouts of adolescents. Telephone the parents of friends whom they say they are visiting. Find ways to limit contact with friends who have behavior problems and promote contact with friends who are a positive influence.

• Talk to the school and suggest similar principles are applied. Request that the school watch for learning problems if you suspect this is a possibility because the frustration experienced by the child with a learning problem may be intolerable for him or her.

Be calm and consistent.

• Set clear house rules and give short, specific commands about the desired behavior, not prohibitions about undesired behavior (eg, "Please walk slowly," rather than "Don't run.").

• Provide consistent, appropriate, and calm consequences for poor behavioral choices.

• When enforcing a rule, avoid getting into arguments or explanations because this merely provides additional attention for the inappropriate behavior.

Create a safety and emergency plan.

• Develop a list of telephone numbers to call in the event that the child's behavior causes a threat to his or her own safety or the safety of others.

• Proactively remove weapons from the home.

• Watch for situations that trigger outbursts.

• Gather the telephone numbers for hotlines, on-call telephone numbers for your pediatrician's practice, or area mental health crisis response team contact information.

Modified from: American Academy of Pediatrics Task Force on Mental Health. *Addresssing Mental Health Concerns in Primary Care: A Clinician's Toolkit* [CD-ROM]. Elk Grove Village, IL: American Academy of Pediatrics; 2010.

Anxiety Disorders: What to Look For

Identifying an anxiety disorder in your child can be difficult not only because his symptoms may be internal, but also because certain signs of anxiety—particularly restlessness and poor concentration—may be misinterpreted as symptoms of ADHD. Children with an anxiety disorder, however, experience more than a general lack of focus or a restless response to boredom. Their anxiety and worry are clear-cut, often focusing on specific situations or thoughts. They may seem tense, irritable, tired, or stressed out. They may not sleep well, and may even experience brief panic attacks—involving a pounding heart, difficulty breathing, nausea, shaking, and intense fears—that occur for no apparent reason. While their school performance may be equivalent to that of children with ADHD alone, they tend to experience a wider variety of social difficulties and have more problems at school than children with ADHD alone. At the same time, they may behave in less disruptive ways than children with ADHD alone because their anxiety may inhibit spontaneous or impulsive behavior. Instead, they may tend to seem inefficient or distracted—having a great deal of difficulty remembering facts or processing concepts or ideas.

Your child can be an important source of information that may lead to a diagnosis of anxiety disorder, although some children are reluctant to admit to any symptoms even if they are quite significant. If the possibility of an anxiety disorder concerns you, be sure to discuss with her any fears or worries she has and listen carefully to her response. Report her comments to her pediatrician and/or psychologist, and encourage her to speak directly with these professionals. In the meantime, ask yourself the following:

- **Did frightening or stressful experiences occur earlier in her life?** Such experiences (for example, loss of a loved one, exposure to violence) can later cause emotional distress, such as post-traumatic stress disorder. Symptoms may resemble symptoms of ADHD.
- **Does she seem excessively worried or anxious about a number of situations or activities (such as peer relationships or school performance)?** Are her fears largely irrational—that is, overly exaggerated or unrealistic—rather than being realistic worries about punishment for negative behavior? Does she find it difficult to control her worrying?

- **Does her anxiety lead to restlessness, fatigue, difficulty concentrating, irritability, muscle tension, and/or sleep disturbance?**
- **Does her anxiety or its outward symptoms significantly impair her social, academic, or other functioning?**
- **Does her anxiety occur more days than not and continue for a significant duration?** Have her anxiety symptoms lasted for at least 6 months? Do her bouts of anxiety occur at least 3 to 5 times per week and last for at least an hour?
- **Is her anxiety unrelated to another disorder, substance abuse, or other identifiable cause?** A child who is distressed over a life event, who is abusing drugs, or whose family is in conflict may exhibit some of the symptoms of anxiety disorder. It is important to consider these other causes as the reason for anxiety instead of a formal anxiety disorder.
- **As a young child, did she experience developmental delays or severe anxiety at being separated from a parent, express frequent or numerous fears, or experience unusual stress?** Children with ADHD and a coexisting anxiety disorder are more likely to have experienced developmental delays in early childhood and more stressful life events such as parental divorce or separation.
- **Have others in her family been diagnosed with anxiety disorders?** Anxiety disorders tend to run in families. A careful review of your family's medical history may provide insight into your child's condition.

These are some symptoms of anxiety disorders, and their presence may indicate a need to have your child evaluated by her pediatrician or mental health provider. The sooner your child is properly treated for anxiety, the sooner she can improve her functioning and balance in her daily life.

Treatment

Treatment for children with ADHD and an anxiety disorder relies on a combination of approaches geared to each child's specific situation—including educating the child and his family about the condition; encouraging ongoing input from school personnel; and initiating behavior therapy, including cognitive-behavioral techniques as well as traditional psychotherapy, family therapy, and medication management.

Behavior therapies are among the most proven and effective non-medication treatments for anxiety disorders. (The effectiveness of traditional psychotherapy has been less well studied.) Behavior therapies target *changing the child's behaviors* caused by the anxiety rather than focusing on the child's internal conflicts. Cognitive-behavioral therapy techniques help children *restructure their thoughts* into a more positive framework so that they can become more assertive and increase their level of positive functioning. For example, a child can learn to identify anxious feelings and thoughts, recognize how his body feels when it responds to anxiety, and devise a plan to mentally cut down on these symptoms when they appear. Other behavioral techniques that can be used for treating anxiety include modeling appropriate behaviors, role-playing, relaxation techniques, and gradual desensitization to the specific experiences that make a given child anxious.

Decisions about medication treatment of ADHD and a coexisting anxiety disorder depend largely on the relative strength of each condition. In the Multimodal Treatment Study of Children with Attention Deficit Hyperactivity Disorder of large numbers of children with ADHD and various coexisting conditions, behavioral treatments were equally as effective as medication treatment for children with ADHD and parent-reported anxiety symptoms. It was not known, however, how many of these children had true anxiety disorders.

In general, if your child's ADHD symptoms impede his functioning more than the anxiety does, and a medication approach is recommended, his pediatrician may choose to begin treating him with stimulants first. As the doctor adjusts your child's dosage for maximal effect, she will monitor your child for side effects such as jitteriness or overfocusing—possible responses to stimulants among children with ADHD and an anxiety disorder. If your child begins taking stimulant medication, his coexisting anxiety symptoms may decrease in some cases, while at the same time there is improvement in the ADHD itself. If those ADHD symptoms do improve with medication and his anxiety diminishes as well, his pediatrician may want to review his diagnosis to reconsider whether the anxiety actually stemmed from the ADHD-related behavior, rather than being a sign of an anxiety disorder. On the other hand, if the ADHD symptoms improve but your child's anxiety remains, his pediatrician may decide to add another type of medication. These medications are often in the class of medications known as selective serotonin reuptake inhibitor (SSRI).

ANXIETY
MEASURES THAT PARENTS CAN TAKE

- Identify your child's worries and fears and set goals for reducing symptoms.
  - Learn strategies to improve coping skills (eg, deep breathing, muscle relaxation, positive self-talk, thought stopping, thinking of a safe place).
  - Ask your physician to recommend material or Web courses that might be helpful.
- One of the best-validated approaches to anxiety and phobias is gradually to increase exposure to the feared objects or experiences. The eventual goal is to master rather than avoid feared things.
  - Start out with brief exposure to the feared object or activity and gradually make it longer.
    - Imagine or talk about the feared object or activity or look at pictures.
    - Learn to tolerate a short exposure.
    - Tolerate a longer exposure in a group or with a coach.
    - Tolerate the feared activity alone but with a chance to get help if needed.
  - During these trials you need to stay as calm and confident as possible. Otherwise, it will be a cue for your child to become distressed.
  - For some children who are vulnerable to anxiety disorder, it is necessary to promptly return them to the anxiety-producing situation. School phobia is an example.
    - Make sure that this avoidance is not due to bullying, trauma, learning difficulties, and medical conditions that may be contributing to stress and fear.
    - Partner with school personnel to manage your child's return to school.
    - Gently but firmly insist that your child attend school, coupled with positive feedback and calm support.
    - If you are uncomfortable with any of these recommendations, seek help from your pediatrician or a mental health specialist.
- Work with your child to rename the fear (ie, "annoying worry") and become its "boss."
- Reward brave behavior.
  - Give positive feedback or small rewards for displaying "brave behavior."
- Pay attention to your own parenting style.
  - Children can become anxious if parents are inconsistent about rules and expectations.
  - Try to eliminate factors that increase anxiety ("I know Dad will get angry if I bring home a bad grade.").
  - Be aware of unrealistic thinking ("I know that the only reason Mom and Dad work hard is so I can go to a better school, so I'm afraid that if I don't do well….").

Modified from: American Academy of Pediatrics Task Force on Mental Health. *Addresssing Mental Health Concerns in Primary Care: A Clinician's Toolkit* [CD-ROM]. Elk Grove Village, IL: American Academy of Pediatrics; 2010.

Mood Disorders

Like anxiety disorders, mood disorders, such as depression and bipolar disorder, often involve subtle, internalized symptoms that can be difficult to recognize until they are expressed in outward behavior. Mood disorders occur in 15% to 20% of children with ADHD. Children with ADHD often have difficulty with irritability, moodiness, and emotional immaturity and tend to overreact to disappointments or frustration. If these problems are severe or interfere with functioning, evaluation for a mood disorder is recommended.

Types of Mood Disorders

The mood disorders most likely to be experienced by children with ADHD include dysthymic disorder, MDD, and bipolar disorder. Dysthymic disorder can be characterized as a chronic low-grade depression, persistent irritability, and a state of demoralization, often with low self-esteem. Major depressive disorder is a more extreme form of depression, often with a more sudden onset, that can occur in children with ADHD and even more frequently among adults with ADHD. Dysthymic disorder and MDD typically develop several years after a child is diagnosed with ADHD and, if left untreated, may worsen over time. Bipolar disorder is a severe mood disorder that has only recently been recognized as occurring in children. Unlike adults who experience distinct periods of elation and significant depression, children with bipolar disorder present a more complex disturbance of extreme emotional instability, behavioral difficulties, and social problems. There is significant overlap with symptoms of ADHD, and many children with bipolar disorder also qualify for a diagnosis of ADHD.

What to Look For

Every child feels discouraged or acts irritable once in a while. Children with ADHD, who so often must deal with extra challenges at school and with peers, may exhibit these behaviors more than most. If your child feels depressed, however, or seems irritable or sad a large portion of each day, more days than not, he may have a coexisting dysthymic disorder. To be diagnosed with dysthymic disorder, a child must also have at least 2 of the following symptoms:

- Poor appetite or overeating
- Insomnia or excessive sleeping
- Low energy or fatigue
- Low self-esteem
- Poor concentration or difficulty making decisions
- Feelings of hopelessness

Before dysthymic disorder can be diagnosed, children must have had these symptoms for a year or longer, although symptoms may have subsided for up to 2 months at a time within that year. The symptoms also must not be caused by another mood disorder, such as MDD or bipolar disorder; a medical condition; substance abuse; or just be related to ADHD itself (low self-esteem stemming from poor functioning in school, for example). Finally, the symptoms must be shown to significantly impair your child's social, academic, or other areas of functioning in daily life.

Major depressive disorder is marked by a nearly constant depressed or irritable mood or a marked loss of interest or pleasure in all or nearly all daily activities. In addition to the symptoms listed previously for dysthymic disorder, a child with MDD may cry daily; withdraw from others; become extremely self-critical; talk about dying; or even think about, plan, or carry out a suicide attempt. Unlike the brief outbursts of temper exhibited by a child with ODD who does not get his way, the irritability of a child with depression may be nearly constant and not linked to any clear cause. His inability to concentrate differs from ADHD-type inattention in that it is accompanied by other symptoms of depression, such as loss of appetite or loss of interest in favorite activities. Finally, the depression itself stems from no apparent cause—as opposed to becoming depressed in response to parental divorce or any other stressful situation. (In fact, research has shown that the intactness of a child's family and its socioeconomic status have little or no effect on whether a child develops MDD.) While children with ADHD/CD alone are not at higher than normal risk for attempting suicide, children with ADHD/CD who also have an MDD and are involved in substance abuse are more likely to make such an attempt and should be carefully watched. Talk of suicide (even if you are not sure whether it is serious), a suicide attempt, self-injury, any violent behavior, or severe withdrawal should be considered an emergency that requires the immediate attention of your child's pediatrician, psychologist, or local hospital.

A depressed child may admit to feeling guilty or sad, or he may deny having any problems. It is important to keep in mind that many depressed children refuse to admit to their feelings, and parents often overlook the subtle behaviors that signal a mood disorder. By keeping in close contact with his teacher, bringing your child to each of his treatment reviews with his pediatrician, and including him in all discussions of his treatment as appropriate to his age, you can improve the chances that his pediatrician or mental health professional will detect any signs of developing depression, and that he will have someone to talk to about his feelings.

A child with bipolar disorder and ADHD is prone to explosive outbursts, extreme mood swings (high, low, or mixed mood), and severe behavioral problems. Chronic irritability can be one of the most prominent features. A child with bipolar disorder is often highly impulsive and aggressive, with prolonged outbursts typically "coming out of nowhere" or in response to trivial frustrations. He may have a history of anxiety. He may also have an extremely high energy level and may experience racing thoughts and inflated self-esteem or grandiosity, extreme talkativeness, physical and emotional agitation, overly sexual behavior, and/or a reduced need for sleep. These symptoms can alternate with periods of depression or irritability, during which his behavior resembles that of a child with MDD. A child with ADHD/bipolar disorder typically has poor social skills. Family relationships are often very strained because of the child's extremely unpredictable, aggressive, or defiant behavior. Early on the symptoms may only occur at home, but often begin to occur in other settings as the child gets older.

Bipolar disorder is a serious psychiatric disorder that can sometimes include psychotic symptoms (delusions/hallucinations) or self-injurious behavior, such as cutting, suicidal thoughts/impulses, and substance abuse. Many children with bipolar disorder have a family history of bipolar disorder, mood disorder, ADHD, and/or substance abuse. Children with ADHD and bipolar disorder are at higher risk than those with ADHD alone for substance abuse and other serious problems during adolescence.

If your child has ADHD with coexisting bipolar disorder, his pediatrician may refer him to a child psychiatrist for further assessment, diagnosis, and recommendations for treatment.

DEPRESSION
SOME USEFUL INFORMATIONAL LINKS

- **American Academy of Child & Adolescent Psychiatry**

  www.aacap.org

- **Guidelines for Adolescent Depression in Primary Care (GLAD-PC): I. Identification, Assessment, and Initial Management**

  http://pediatrics.aappublications.org/cgi/content/full/120/5/e1299

- **Guidelines for Adolescent Depression in Primary Care (GLAD-PC): II. Treatment and Ongoing Management**

  http://pediatrics.aappublications.org/cgi/content/full/120/5/e1313

- **GLAD-PC Tool Kit**

  www.thereachinstitute.org/files/document/GLAD-PCToolkit.pdf

- **Hawaii State Department of Health, Child and Adolescent Mental Health Division, Evidence Based Services, Intervention and Treatment Tools**

  http://hawaii.gov

  This Web page has links to charts of evidence-based child and adolescent psychosocial interventions and evidence-based child and adolescent psychopharmacology.

- **US Preventive Health Services Task Force, Major Depressive Disorder in Children and Adolescents**

  www.ahrq.gov/CLINIC/uspstf/uspschdepr.htm

Treatment

As with ADHD with anxiety disorders, treatment of ADHD with depression usually involves a broad approach. Treatment approaches may include a combination of cognitive-behavioral therapy, interpersonal therapy (focusing on areas of grief, interpersonal relationships, disputes, life transitions, and personal difficulties), and traditional psychotherapy (to help with self-understanding, identification of feelings, improving self-esteem, changing patterns of behavior, interpersonal interactions, and coping with conflicts), as well as family therapy when needed.

Medication management approaches, as with ADHD and other coexisting conditions, include treating the most disabling condition first. If your child's ADHD-related symptoms are causing most of his functioning problems, or the signs of depression are not completely clear, your child's pediatrician is likely to start with stimulant medication to treat the ADHD. In cases when the depressive symptoms turn out to stem from poor functioning due to ADHD and not to a depressive disorder, they may diminish as the ADHD symptoms improve. If the symptoms of ADHD and depression improve, your child's pediatrician will probably maintain stimulant treatment alone. If his ADHD symptoms improve but his depression remains the same, even after a reasonable trial of the type of broad psychotherapeutic approach described previously, his pediatrician may add another medication, most commonly an SSRI—a class of medications including fluoxetine (Prozac), citalopram (Celexa), sertraline (Zoloft), paroxetine (Paxil), and fluvoxamine (Luvox). These SSRIs can make the symptoms of bipolar disorder worse, so a careful evaluation must be completed before starting medication. If this approach is unsuccessful, you may be referred to a developmental/behavioral pediatrician or a psychiatrist, who may try other classes of medications.

DEPRESSION
MEASURES THAT PARENTS CAN TAKE

Encourage Healthy Habits
- These include exercise, outdoor play, healthy diet, sleep, limiting screen time, one-on-one time with parents, praise for positive behavior, and acknowledgment of the child's strengths. Caring for oneself can be honestly presented as therapeutic.

Consider the Environment
- **Think about whether there are grief and loss issues in your child and/or other family members.** Grief and loss are virtually universal childhood experiences. Children vary widely in their reactions to these events, depending on their developmental level, temperament, prior state of mental health, coping mechanisms, parents' responses, and support system. Seek supportive counseling if this does not seem to be resolving appropriately.
- **Reduce stress.** Your family can work to try to reduce stresses and increase support for your child/ adolescent. This may involve reasonable and short-term changes in demands and responsibilities, including negotiating extensions or other ways of reducing stress at school; it can also include seeking help for others in the family who are distressed. If you as a parent are grieving a loss or manifesting symptoms of depression, it is particularly important that you address your own needs and find additional support for your child and other family members.
- **Guns should be removed from the home and other weapons, medications (including over-the-counter preparations and acetaminophen), and alcohol should be removed from the home, destroyed, or secured.**

DEPRESSION

MEASURES THAT PARENTS CAN TAKE (CONTINUED)

Educate Your Family

- Your child is not making the symptoms up.

- What looks like laziness or crossness can be symptoms of depression.

- There is often a family history of depression; talking about this may reduce stigma and increase empathy in other family members.

- Depression is very common and not the result of lack of coping ability or personal strength.

- The hopelessness of depression is a symptom, not an accurate reflection of reality. However, this negative view of the world and of future possibilities can be hard to penetrate.

- Treatment works, though it can take several weeks for improvement, and the affected individual is often the last person to recognize that it has taken place.

Help Your Child to Develop Cognitive and Coping Skills

- Many negative thoughts can be empathetically challenged and looked at from another perspective. Helpful metaphors include, "Little steps uphill, big steps downhill"; "Long journeys start with a single step"; "The glass is half full, not half empty."

- Relaxation techniques and visualization (eg, practicing relaxing cued by a pleasant memory, imagining being in a pleasant place) can be helpful for sleep and for anxiety-provoking situations.

- Take advantage of what your child already does to feel better or relax and, if appropriate, encourage more of that (behavioral activation). Encourage a focus on strengths rather than weaknesses. Encourage doing more of what the teen is good at.

Help Your Child to Develop Problem-Solving Skills

- Determine what small, achievable steps would help your child feel that he or she is on the way to overcoming his or her problems.

- Suggest that your child begin to list out difficulties, prioritize them, and concentrate efforts on one issue one small step at a time.

Rehearse Behavior and Social Skills

- Reactions to particular situations or people often seem to trigger or maintain low mood. If these can be identified, assist your child in developing and practicing means of avoidance or alternative responses.

- Encourage your child to practice doing things and thinking thoughts that improve mood.

<table>
<tr><td align="center">**DEPRESSION**
MEASURES THAT PARENTS CAN TAKE (CONTINUED)</td></tr>
</table>

Create a Safety and Emergency Plan

- Develop a list of telephone numbers to call in the event of a sudden increase in distress.
- Remove weapons and other potentially lethal products from your home.
- Watch for risk factors for suicide, such as increased agitation, stressors, loss of rational thinking, and expressed wishes to die.
- If your child is starting a medication for depression, develop a monitoring schedule with her physician.
- Locate numbers for suicide or depression hotlines, on-call telephone numbers for your physician, or contact information for the area mental health crisis response team.

Modified from: American Academy of Pediatrics Task Force on Mental Health. *Addresssing Mental Health Concerns in Primary Care: A Clinician's Toolkit* [CD-ROM]. Elk Grove Village, IL: American Academy of Pediatrics; 2010.

Tics, Tourette Disorder, and Obsessive-Compulsive Disorder

Tics are rapid, repetitive movements or vocal utterances. They may be motor (like excessive eye blinking) or vocal (such as a habitual cough or chronic repetitive throat-clearing noises), chronic (continuing throughout childhood), or transient (lasting less than 1–2 years). In children who eventually develop tic disorders and ADHD, the ADHD usually develops 2 to 3 years before the tics.

Tourette disorder, which is quite rare, is a more severe form of tic disorder involving motor and vocal tics that occur many times per day. The average age at which it appears is 7 years. While children with Tourette disorder may develop ADHD, the 2 disorders are separate and independent conditions. Attention-deficit/hyperactivity disorder is not a variant of Tourette disorder, nor is Tourette disorder just a variety of ADHD. Research has shown that chronic tic disorders, Tourette disorder, and OCD may stem from some common factors, and a child with any of these conditions is quite likely to also have ADHD.

Obsessive-compulsive disorder involves such symptoms as obsessive thoughts (such as a highly exaggerated fear of germs) and compulsive behaviors (for example, excessive hand-washing in an attempt to reduce the fear of germs) that the child is unable to control or limit.

In this sense, OCD is similar to tic disorders and Tourette disorder, and creates additional functioning problems for children with ADHD.

What to Look For

Tics tend to resemble certain ADHD-related symptoms—fidgeting and making random noises in particular—and may occasionally be mistaken for signs of ADHD. True tics, however, differ from ADHD-type fidgetiness or hyperactivity in that they almost always involve rapid, repeated, identical movements of the face or shoulders, or vocal sounds or phrases that may cause a child to become socially isolated. The diagnosis of Tourette disorder is made only when the tics developed before 18 years of age include motor and vocal tics, occur many times each day, and continue for at least a year. Though the intensity of the tics may increase or decrease periodically, a child with active Tourette disorder is rarely completely tic-free for more than 3 months at a time. Tourette disorder may also resolve by itself, without any explanation.

While tic disorders and Tourette disorder involve outbursts of simple movements or vocalizations, OCD consists of obsessive thoughts and compulsive behaviors. In contrast to the common childhood "obsessions" with computer games or television, OCD-type obsessive thoughts and behaviors provide no pleasure and stem from no rational desire or motivation. Rather, they occur because the child is unable to stop them, even when he realizes that they are inappropriate—and they can interfere with his functioning for literally hours a day.

Treatment

Mild or transient tics may not need to be treated with any medication. In the past, stimulant medications were not recommended for children with ADHD and a coexisting tic disorder because the stimulants were thought to be a possible cause of Tourette disorder. It is now known that starting stimulants does not cause Tourette disorder or even increase tics in most children with ADHD. Stimulants may actually result in improvements in the tics in some cases. However, stimulants at high doses may bring out or exaggerate tics in a child with ADHD, who would have eventually developed them even without stimulants. The potential disadvantage of mildly increased tics is often outweighed by the effectiveness of stimulants in treating the symptoms of ADHD. Meanwhile, lowering the stimulant dose or switching to a different medication can sometimes decrease or eliminate some tics altogether. If your child's tics are especially severe or socially disruptive, a combination of stimulants and clonidine, guanfacine, or other medications, such as risperidone, may also be considered. Possible side effects must be taken into account when using any of these medications.

Learning, Motor Skills, and Communication Disorders

Most learning problems encountered by children with ADHD are not due to learning disabilities. About 40% of children with ADHD experience learning challenges, such as work production problems and organizing difficulties, that are categorized as learning "problems," not disabilities. Learning disabilities are generally thought of as a child's failure to develop specific academic skills at the expected level in spite of adequate intelligence and education. Attention-deficit/hyperactivity disorder itself is not a learning disorder—with proper treatment and support, many children with ADHD can perform as well as their peers academically. The true incidence of coexisting learning disabilities is not clear because of discrepancies in how they are defined, and estimates vary widely.

Although there is increasing controversy about how learning disorders should be defined, they have been defined in the past by showing that there is a significant discrepancy between a child's cognitive abilities, as measured by standard IQ tests, and his actual learning, as measured on individually administered achievement tests in reading, math, and written expression. The problems with this "discrepancy" model are that few characteristics differentiate poor readers whose skills differ from those predicted by their IQ scores from those whose skills match their IQ scores. In addition, the amount of difference between IQ scores and measured achievement in reading is not necessarily related to the severity of the learning disability, and does not predict the potential for gaining from reading interventions, the reading level of a child over time, or how a child will respond to any given reading program. Using a discrepancy model, children with low average IQs and commensurate low average achievement would not qualify for services, in spite of the evidence that they can equally benefit.

Nonverbal learning disabilities (NLDs) are not generally included in the standard defini-tions of learning disability, but are important to consider, especially when children have coexisting problems with attention. Nonverbal learning disabilities are characterized by a specific pattern of relative strengths and weaknesses in academic skills. This includes well-developed single-word reading and spelling relative to mechanical math. It also presents with weaknesses in social skill areas. Children with NLDs make more efficient use of verbal than nonverbal information in social situations, and thus have difficulty reading social cues. Other recognized disabilities that can interfere with academic functioning include motor skills disorder (developmental coordination disorder) and communication disorders.

Before 2004, a child was not offered services unless there was a discrepancy between abilities (IQ): oral expression, listening comprehension, written expression, basic reading skill, read-ing comprehension, math calculation, and/or math reasoning. This meant, however, that students would have to fail for long periods before they showed sufficiently large delays in academic achievement to satisfy the "severe discrepancy" requirement and begin receiving special education services. This discrepancy requirement was particularly problematic for students living in poverty, students of culturally different backgrounds, or those whose native language was not English. In 2004 the law was revised, and school districts are not required to use the discrepancy model to show that a student has a specific learning disabil-ity. Schools can now use measures that are more relevant to the instruction students receive in the classroom. Now school districts can determine if a student responds to scientifically based interventions as a part of the evaluation procedures. Response to intervention (RTI) is an example of this kind of process. In RTI, students who show signs of learning difficulties are provided with a series of increasingly intensive, individualized instructional or behavioral interventions.

DISORDERS THAT INTERFERE WITH ACADEMIC FUNCTIONING

Learning Disorders

- Reading disorder
- Mathematics disorder
- Disorder of written expression
- Nonverbal learning disability*

Motor Skills Disorder

- Developmental coordination disorder

Communication Disorders

- Expressive language disorder (difficulties with using language to express oneself, including having a limited amount of speech, limited range of vocabulary, difficulty acquiring new words, using appropriate grammar, etc)
- Mixed receptive-expressive language disorder (difficulty understanding and using language, words, sentences, or specific types of words)
- Phonologic disorder (difficulty with pronunciation or articulation of speech sounds)
- Stuttering

Medical Disorders

- Hearing deficits
- Vision deficits
- Chronic illnesses

*Not included in the formal *Diagnostic and Statistical Manual of Mental Disorders, Fourth Edition, Text Revision* diagnostic categories, 2000.

Learning Disorders

Reading Disorders

Reading disorders, the most common and best studied of the learning disabilities, account for 80% of all children diagnosed as learning disabled. Children with reading disorders are able to visualize letters and words but have difficulty recognizing that letters and combinations of letters represent different sounds. Most reading disorders involve difficulties with recognizing single words rather than with reading comprehension. The cause often lies in the area of the child's "phonologic awareness"—difficulty perceiving how sounds make up words. Reading disorders—even including letter reversals—have little to do with vision. These problems make it quite difficult for children to add new words to their reading reper- toire and become good readers. While their listening and speaking skills may be adequate, they may have trouble naming objects (such as quickly coming up with the word for "com- puter" or "backpack") and/or remembering verbal sequences (such as "The boy saw the man who was driving the red car."). A smaller group of children also have reading disabilities that involve comprehension, and these children tend to have poor receptive language skills—that is, difficulty understanding language even when it is spoken to them. A reading disorder, depending on how it is defined, is not necessarily a lifelong condition, but these problems do persist into adulthood in at least 40% of children.

Like all other learning disabilities, reading disorders cannot be detected through neurologic tests, such as special examinations, electroencephalograms (EEGs: brain wave tests), or brain scans like computed tomography and magnetic resonance imaging. They are identified when a child's reading level or language achievement scores are significantly lower than those of his classmates. In assessing reading disabilities, it is important to identify each component of your child's problem so that specific treatment measures can be applied. It is also important to address the attentional and behavioral aspects of the ADHD so that your child can make optimal progress at school.

Mathematics Disorder

Mathematics disorder can be thought of as a type of learning disability in which spoken language is not affected, but computational math is. Children with mathematics disorder also may have difficulties with motor and spatial, organizational, and social skills. Children with coexisting ADHD, or even ADHD alone, can have additional problems in math—such as delays in committing math facts to memory, the making of careless math errors, rushing through problems and impulsively putting down the wrong answers or not showing their work, and making errors because they misaligned columns during addition or long division. Although math disabilities are about as common as reading disabilities, they are not well studied. It is not known whether math skills stem from the innate abilities of children to understand the concepts of magnitude or quantities and compare numbers, or whether they arise in brain areas that are responsible for language, visual-spatial, or attention and

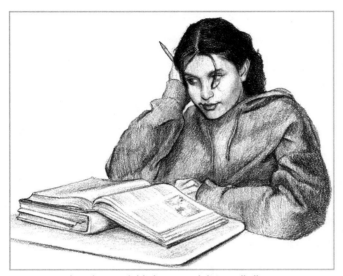

Being in touch with your child's learning abilities will allow you to provide the support she needs in order to succeed in the classroom.

memory systems. It is generally agreed that children with mathematics disability have a deficit in recalling math facts. Accurate and fluent recall of single digit math facts is felt to be important in freeing up higher brain areas for learning and applying more complex tasks. Children with both reading and math disabilities struggle particularly with word problem-solving.

Written Expression Disorder

Children with written expression disorder can have difficulty composing sentences and paragraphs; organizing paragraphs; using correct grammar, punctuation, and spelling in their written work; and writing legibly. Children with spoken-language problems can develop problems with written language as well as math. Children with ADHD can also have difficulty with taking the mental time to plan their writing, and their handwriting can be immature and sometimes unreadable without necessarily having a written expression disorder. When handwriting problems are more a function of ADHD than a written expression or motor skills disorder, they sometimes improve rapidly and dramatically with appropriate stimulant medication treatment.

Nonverbal Learning Disability

Nonverbal learning disability is a condition that is not yet formally categorized as a disorder but that has been the subject of increasing interest. It is particularly important to consider in children with ADHD because it relates to attentional functioning. It is often difficult to decide whether a child with ADHD has a coexisting NLD or whether he just has an NLD that mimics ADHD—especially the inattentive symptoms.

Nonverbal learning disability accounts for about 5% to 10% of children with learning disabilities. It consists of a cluster of deficits, including poor visuospatial skills, problems with social skills, and impaired math ability. Problems with disorganization, inconsistent school performance, and social problems may lead to an evaluation for ADHD. In some cases this makes children with NLD difficult to differentiate from children with Asperger disorder. General functioning in children with NLD younger than 4 years can be relatively typical or only involve mild deficits. Following this period, children can develop disruptive behavior and may develop hyperactivity and inattention. They are frequently thought of as acting out and hyperactive, and are commonly identified by their teachers as overtalkative, trouble makers, or behavior problems. As they grow older, their high activity level can disappear. By older childhood and early adolescence, problems can tend to be more internal, characterized by withdrawal, anxiety, depression, unusual behaviors, and social skills problems. Interactions with other children may become more difficult, and their faces can seem unexpressive. These behaviors can be accompanied by deficits in how they judge social situations, judgment, and interaction skills. Children with NLD are particularly prone to emotional problems over the course of their development, as opposed to children with other learning disabilities. Nonverbal learning disabilities are less prevalent than language-based learning disorders. Where it is estimated that about 4% to 20% of the general population have identifiable learning disabilities, it is thought that only 1% to 10% of those individuals would be found to have NLD.

Children with NLD are often not identified until late elementary school or middle school, when the peer problems increase and academic tasks become more complicated. They frequently develop symptoms of depression and anxiety.

Academic Problems

As was pointed out earlier in this chapter, children with ADHD frequently experience significant challenges at school and elsewhere that cannot be formally categorized as disabilities or formal disorders. Forty percent of children with ADHD, for example, who do not qualify for a diagnosis of learning disability still experience learning problems that lead to underachievement at school. These learning problems may include

- Inattention and distractibility
- Lack of persistence and inconsistent performance
- A tendency to become easily bored or to rush through or not complete work
- Impulsive responses and careless errors
- Difficulty self-correcting mistakes
- A limited ability to sit still and listen
- Difficulty with time-limited tasks and test taking
- Problems with planning, homework flow, and work completion
- Difficulty taking notes or performing other forms of multitasking
- Difficulty memorizing facts
- Difficulty organizing and producing written work
- Immature and slow handwriting that can also create obstacles in expressive writing
- Difficulty with reading comprehension

Stimulant medications that decrease your child's ADHD symptoms are likely to help her address many of these problems. Behavior therapy techniques aimed at increasing or decreasing specific behaviors at home and in school can also prove beneficial. As discussed in chapters 5 and 7, specific behavioral goals, such as improving completion of assignments, can be addressed by understanding your child's individual strengths and weaknesses and collaborating with school staff in using positive reinforcement, appropriate behavioral techniques, daily report cards, and ongoing monitoring.

Motor Skills Disorder

Motor skills disorder, also known as developmental coordination disorder, is diagnosed when motor skills problems significantly interfere with academic achievement or activities of daily living. It is frequently overlooked in children with ADHD due to its nonspecific cluster of symptoms—yet it can affect children's lives by interfering with writing and other academic activities or preventing children from participating at their classmates' level in sports and play. Children with ADHD and other learning disabilities frequently have motor skills disorder as well. Motor skills disorder involves a developmental delay of movement and posture that leaves children with coordination substantially below that of others of their age and intelligence level. These children seem so clumsy and awkward they are rarely picked for teams at school. As the years pass, they tend to fall further behind in terms of motor skills, and their confidence diminishes as a result. By adolescence, most children with motor skills disorder not only perform poorly in physical education classes, but may also have a poor physical self-image and perform below expectations academically.

Motor skills disorder may be first identified when a preschooler or kindergartner is unable to perform age-appropriate skills, such as buttoning buttons and catching a ball, or when an elementary school child struggles with writing or sports activities. A child with motor skills disorder may have difficulty with the mechanics of writing, with planning motor actions, or with memorizing motor patterns. While many young children with ADHD but no motor skills disorder may seem clumsy in their younger years, their awkwardness is related more to inattentiveness or impulsivity than to poor motor control and it is frequently outgrown. However, a child with ADHD and coexisting motor skills disorder may not outgrow his clumsiness.

If your child is diagnosed with developmental coordination disorder, he may be referred to a pediatric occupational therapist for individualized therapy and, particularly if his deficits negatively affect his academic performance or daily skills, be recommended for special gym activities at school to promote hand-eye coordination and motor development and improve specific skills.

Communication Disorders

Communication disorders—conditions that interfere with communications with others in everyday life—involve not only the ability to appreciate language sounds (phonologic awareness) but also to acquire, recall, and use vocabulary (semantics) and to deal with word order and appropriately form or comprehend sentences (syntax). Subcategories of these disorders have been identified, including expressive language disorder, mixed receptive-expressive disorder, phonologic disorder, articulation (word pronunciation) disorder, and stuttering.

Because there is such a close association between communication and social relationships, these language deficits are often accompanied by social skills difficulties. Children with ADHD without a language disorder may also have difficulties in using language, particularly in social situations. You may notice that your child has problems with excessive talking, frequent interruption, not listening to what is said, blurting out answers before questions are finished, and having disorganized conversations.

Treatment

Treatments for learning disabilities that lead to strong outcomes include learning strategies (referred to as a cognitive approach), changing learning behaviors (cognitive-behavioral approach), and breaking down tasks into smaller teachable units (task analytic methods). Cognitive strategies target processes that are directly linked to academic skills and encourage academic strategies. Cognitive models target information-processing abilities, such as using memory, as well as developing skill directly linked to academics, such as awareness of how words are constructed (phonologic awareness). Cognitive-behavioral approaches combine these approaches with behavioral principles used during teacher-directed instruction. Cognitive-behavioral strategies help students with self-regulation and forming positive attitudes about themselves and their academic capabilities while they also master strategies that form the basis for effective academic performance. Effective direct instruction methods emphasize providing a student with well-specified learning objectives and detailed sequences of instructional steps. However, if too much class time is spent dealing with behaviors and self-regulation issues, little academic learning will occur because there is no time to teach the academic content. When students are "pulled out" for academic instruction this can obviously pose problems of coming back into the classroom and not understanding what the class is doing. It is very important to carefully balance pull-out activities with the need to acquire this academic content being taught in the classroom.

Children with a learning, motor skills, or communication disability may require tutoring, an in-class aide or other classroom support, an altered curriculum, special education classes, pull-out time, speech-language therapy, occupational therapy, or adaptive physical education. Many children with ADHD benefit from a positive behavior management plan. As described in Chapter 7, many of these services must be provided free of charge by your school district if your child qualifies for coverage by the Individuals with Disabilities Act or Section 504. Your child's pediatrician can also refer your child to private sources for evaluation and help.

While stimulant medication does not improve the academic achievement of children with learning disabilities alone, it can help children who have both learning disabilities and ADHD improve their reading performance and seatwork completion by helping them improve their attention and focus during these tasks. This is most likely due to stimulants' positive effect on children's attentiveness, which allows them to benefit more from special tutoring and other forms of therapy. Thus use of stimulants to treat ADHD symptoms is often recommended as an important part of treatment for ADHD/learning disabilities.

Intellectual Disability

Most forms of intellectual disability (formerly called mental retardation) are recognized early in a child's life, as the child fails to achieve standard developmental milestones at appropriate ages. However, at early ages, developmental delays do not necessarily predict that intellectual disabilities will be present when a child reaches school age. A given child's predicted abilities (IQ) can start to be measured in school-aged children. Whereas an average IQ is around 100, intellectual disabilities are diagnosed in the 2% to 3% of children who score the lowest on a standard IQ test and are delayed to the same extent in such life skills as self-care, self-direction, and the use of academic skills. Eighty-five percent of children with intellectual disability fall into the mild range, with IQ scores from 70 to 55. Intellectual disabilities are often suspected within the first few years of life if children are experiencing lags in the rate of their development in social, self-help, motor skills, and language development. Children with milder forms of intellectual disability may escape detection until their school years, when parents or teachers begin to wonder if their difficulties in learning signal the presence of ADHD or learning disabilities and bring them to a pediatrician for evaluation. In the past, physicians did not believe that ADHD occurred in children with intellectual disabilities. As a result, treatments for ADHD, including stimulant medications, were rarely used to treat children who actually had ADHD and coexisting intellectual disabilities. But recent research reveals that as many as 25% to 40% of children with intellectual disability also have ADHD—significantly more than in the general population.

Treatment for children with intellectual disability includes family support; family education and counseling; special educational programs; paying attention to transitional needs and educational rights; identifying community supports and support groups (such as The Arc); and paying close attention to your child's strengths, abilities, and self-esteem.

Autism Spectrum Disorders (Autism, Asperger, and Related Disorders)

Autism spectrum disorders, also known as PPDs, are characterized by (1) significant deficits in social understanding, (2) delays in communication and unusual use of language, and (3) unusual restricted and repetitive interests or behaviors. In recent years there has been a significant increase in the number of cases reported. The latest estimate of prevalence of ASDs is 1 child in 110. Schools can designate children as qualifying for services under the category of ASDs, although a significant number of children identified for these services do not have an ASD diagnosis by stricter medical standards. About half of children with autism also have intellectual disabilities. The causes of the apparent growing increase in prevalence of ASDs is not known. However, there is no scientific evidence that it is caused by immunizations or mercury, 2 common publicly held notions. Adherence to these theories can significantly undermine vaccination programs that have saved millions of lives.

The number of children with ASDs and ADHD is difficult to determine because children with ASDs alone often have elements of attention problems, impulsiveness, and hyperactivity. A child with an ASD may also have intellectual disability, but even if he does not, his challenges associated with an ASD are likely to prevent him from participating fully socially and in many school and home activities. The most severe form of ASDs, autistic disorder (autism), involves severe language and social impairment and abnormal, repetitive, and unusual patterns of behavior. Autistic disorder usually becomes manifest by age 3 years. Children with autism are unable to form typical social relationships with others. Coexisting ADHD can add a significant overlay of aggressive, impulsive, or hyperactive symptoms to the behavior of a child with autism, although it is not always easy to separate the ADHD behaviors from those related to the autism itself.

Children with Asperger disorder are of average to above-average intelligence and are able to function adequately in many aspects of daily life. They do not have a history of language delays but have difficulty making conversation and using polite manners, and may have an unusual tone of voice. They experience significant disabilities in social interaction with peers and display unusually intense and narrow interests or obsessions. It is sometimes difficult to differentiate children with Asperger disorder from those with NLD, as mentioned previously. Children with Asperger disorder may have coexisting ADHD and are at increased risk of developing anxiety or depressive disorders. In the future, it is likely that the diagnosis of Asperger disorder will be discontinued, and diagnosis of high-functioning autism will replace it.

Treatment

Individualized educational programming, behavior therapy, and family support are essential elements in the treatment of children with ASDs. Identifying children with ASDs early is critical because intensive early intervention (20 hours per week or more) can lead to very significant gains in connecting with the social world and developing language, communication, and cognitive skills. Medication may be helpful for specific symptoms. Stimulants can usually be used to treat ADHD symptoms in children with combined ASDs and ADHD, although the rates of side effects and nonresponse are somewhat greater than in those with ADHD alone. Many children with ASDs/ADHD may need special education–related services, such as speech-language therapy and behavior management programs. (See Chapter 7 for descriptions of resources and laws relating to student disabilities.)

You can further support your child's progress by educating yourself about his condition, monitoring the latest research on his areas of disability, and advocating for his rights and appropriate services within the public school system (see Chapter 7).

Coexisting Problems

Children with ADHD may have problems in some of the areas described previously, even though they fall short of receiving formal diagnoses in these areas. You should not hesitate to confer with your child's pediatrician, teachers, mental health professionals, and community support agencies to seek help even if your child falls short or receiving a formal diagnosis. Not having a formal diagnosis certainly does not mean that no help is needed.

Recognizing Coexisting Strengths

Finally, but *most* importantly, don't forget to pay attention to your child's coexisting strengths. The main focus should always be on your child, and not on his challenges, disabilities, and coexisting conditions. Children with ADHD frequently meet with disapproval, social rejection, and other forms of discouragement. However, if encouraged to grow up aware of and invested in their own talents, strengths, positive energy, and achievements, they can mature with a healthy and balanced perspective and better self-esteem as they head toward productive and successful adult lives.

Chapter 10

Complementary and Alternative Treatments for ADHD

In this book you have been introduced to the treatment approaches that have been proven most effective for children with attention-deficit/hyperactivity disorder (ADHD). You are also likely to read or hear about complementary and alternative treatments. In this chapter we will define and discuss these treatments.

Complementary treatments are meant to be used in conjunction with the multimodal treatments already discussed in this book. They are added to the usual effective medication and/or sound psychosocial/behavioral treatments. They are often used by parents for children who have not experienced sufficient improvement despite standard treatments or who have symptoms not addressed by the primary treatments, such as irritability or mood swings. They are also used by parents who want to enhance their child's overall health and well-being while they are treating the child for ADHD.

Alternative treatments are those that claim to be as effective, or more effective, than prescription medications and the scientifically sound psychosocial/behavioral treatments for the core symptoms of ADHD that you have read about. These types of treatment are often used by parents for children who have not experienced sufficient improvement in spite of standard treatments, who are uncomfortable with the idea of daily medication use, or who want to explore all possible avenues of treatment for their child. Some of these treatments have the additional attraction of being proposed as "cures" or "natural treatments." The theories on which they are based may make a great deal of intuitive sense as well—for example, when they target a child's diet to treat hyperactivity or his hearing to help attention. The question with these treatments, as with more traditional treatments is whether they have been shown to reliably produce positive and sustained effects for most children with ADHD. Some have actually been proven ineffective. Others may or may not eventually be demonstrated to have a positive effect, but have not yet been studied sufficiently for their use to be recommended at this time.

Because the claims for ADHD treatments are so vast and so varied, it is important to sub-ject any report of a new or unconventional treatment approach to the same scrutiny and consideration you would apply to any major decision affecting your family: by considering the source of the information, the reasonableness of its claims, and the scientific evidence that backs them up, and by discussing the treatment with experts in the field such as your child's pediatrician or psychologist. In this chapter you will learn how to consider the validity of claims for ADHD treatments by

- Knowing what target behaviors the proposed treatment claims to address
- Understanding how a proposed treatment is scientifically evaluated, and what steps must be taken to prove that a treatment is sound
- Reviewing the evidence for and against proposed ADHD treatments, such as dietary changes; visual, auditory, and sensory integration approaches; hypnotherapy; biofeed-back; applied kinesiology; homeopathy; and various other methods
- Considering the types of questions you should ask, and the steps you should take, before committing effort, time, and money to a new form of treatment, however promising it may seem

As part of your consideration of any measure, you might see if evidence is available on a given treatment from the National Center for Complementary and Alternative Medicine at the National Institutes of Health. Some of this information is contained on their Web site at www.nccam.nih.gov. You might also want to inquire whether a particular treatment will be reimbursed through your health insurance.

How Treatments Are Proven Effective

You may have noticed that the media seem to report on a new treatment for ADHD fre-quently. If so, you may wonder why so many alternative treatments exist for ADHD, and why they so easily gain credibility with the general public. One reason is that, as opposed to such medical conditions as diabetes, the results of a given treatment for ADHD are difficult to measure objectively—that is, there is no blood, urine, or other laboratory test that can prove conclusively that the treatment has worked. Instead, as you will see, the effectiveness of treatments for ADHD are judged through rigorous studies of groups undergoing the treatment compared with those who are not. Because effects of these treatments are determined through relatively subjective methods, such as changes in teachers' and parents' observations, and ratings of behaviors over time—not by objective blood, urine, or magnetic resonance imaging studies—it is often more difficult, even with careful statistical analysis, to clearly establish that any proposed standard or alternative treatment for ADHD is well-founded. If a treatment cannot quickly and objectively be proven effective, it is easier for its proponents to just claim that it works. Thus claims for a particular approach can be greatly exaggerated and widely disseminated long before it has been sufficiently studied.

Yet there is a standard, reliable process for deciding whether a new treatment is effective. This process is called the scientific method, and through it investigators can subject any treatment approach to a reliable series of tests or studies to evaluate its effectiveness. There is a great deal written these days about "evidence-based medicine," which is a set of procedures, resources, and information tools for appraising the strength of the scientific evidence

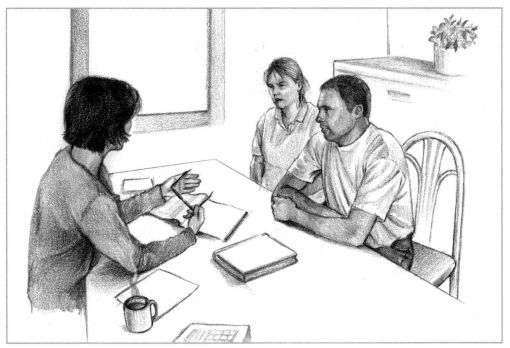

If you do become interested in using complementary and alternative treatments, be sure to discuss your plans first with your child's doctor.

to assist practitioners in applying research findings to the care of individual patients. The medical community now expects treatments strongly recommended for the treatment of ADHD to meet these standards of evidence-based medicine. Studies of treatments for ADHD conducted according to the scientific method make use of research tools, including structured observations, rating scales, and objective tests of the child's functioning, whenever possible. They are structured so that extraneous factors that might influence results are taken into account and designed so that they can be reproduced by other researchers to make sure similar results are achieved.

According to the scientific method and evidence-based medicine, we can only rely on the results of studies relating to a particular treatment if the researchers have

- **Formulated a clear hypothesis.** The researcher must state what she wants to determine through the study. For instance, she might state the hypothesis, "Because diet and nutrition are known to affect brain development, a diet fortified with extra vitamins will have a positive effect on ADHD symptoms." This then will be proved or disproved by a well-conducted study.

- **Created a detailed plan to test the hypothesis.** The researcher must then define the nature of the treatment (for example, state which vitamins will be administered, at what dose, and how frequently), how it will be administered (by parents, by a physician, by the children themselves), how it will be monitored (by counting the number of pills left in the bottle at the end of the study), and how the effects will be measured (through a daily dosage checklist, parents' reports, physicians' records, teacher observations, etc). In this way, the study results can be systematically explained (perhaps it did not work because the children reported taking the vitamins but did not always do so, for example), and other researchers can confirm the results by using the same methods with different sets of children.

- **Defined the group to be tested.** This is an important and sometimes difficult part of creating a reliable study. Can a child be allowed to participate in the study solely on the basis of whether he looks hyperactive to the researchers? Must he have been diagnosed by his pediatrician? Or have the researchers made their own diagnosis according to rigorous research criteria? The group under study must also be large enough for the treatment results to apply to the population as a whole—1, 6, or even 100 children may not be enough, depending on the research question. The group receiving the treatment must be compared with a group not receiving the treatment, and/or another group or groups receiving a different type of treatment for ADHD. The members of the groups under study should otherwise be as similar as possible, and children who might be affected by extraneous influences, such as coexisting disorders, high or low extremes in intelligence, and unusual family circumstances, are sometimes screened out. Depending on the question to be answered, the researcher must limit as many other variables as possible, aside from the treatment under study.

- **Eliminated the power of suggestion.** One way to test whether a treatment is effective is to compare the proposed treatment with a placebo treatment. People often tend to respond to placebos—inactive medications or treatments they believe may work—whether or not the treatment is actually effective in the long run. A person with a headache who is given a "sugar pill," believing it is pain medication, may report that the headache is gone a short time later. In many studies placebos can be shown to be somewhat or very effective. One way to test whether a treatment for ADHD is effective, for example, is to make sure that the subjects do not know whether they are really receiving the proposed treatment or a placebo treatment. In the vitamin treatment example, then, half of the subjects in the study might receive actual megavitamins and the other half would receive an inactive, neutral, but identical-looking pill. Depending on the type of investigation, the study design may work even better if used in a "double-blind" experiment—that is, if the subject, his family, his teacher, and the researcher do not know whether the actual pill or a placebo was used in a particular patient until the study has ended. That way there is no danger that the researcher has inadvertently communicated this information to the subject, his family, or teacher, or that he misinterpreted the results because of what he knew. Of course, if the treatment has specific effects, such as an unusual taste difficult to mimic in the placebo, it may be impossible to keep everyone in the dark about which person got the experimental treatment.

Placebo treatments are more difficult to create when the treatment involves a procedure, such as psychotherapy, rather than a pill. Still, researchers must make every effort to make the real treatment and the placebo treatment equally convincing to the subject.

Having independent evaluators who are unaware of the treatment being used, called blinded, to whether the treatment is the megavitamin or the placebo preparation improves the accuracy of the study.

- **Provided a valid means of evaluating the results.** Some treatment results are easier to evaluate than others. As you've already read, in the case of ADHD, results can be difficult to judge because they cannot be measured through precise laboratory tests or other fully objective measures. Still, researchers can standardize test results through such techniques as quantifying behaviors (having teachers report how many times per day a child interrupted a conversation, got out of his seat without permission, or failed to hear someone talking to him), using standard rating scales, comparing the study subjects' performance to that of the other groups in the study who received different treatments, and measuring changes in the behaviors being studied at predetermined intervals throughout the course of the investigation. Treatments can be evaluated by standardized tests (such as performance on standardized math tests), as well as in terms of the child's performance in the real world (measures of classroom behavior or improvements in family relationships). Rigorous statistical techniques are then used to find any significant differences in results among the groups in the study. The methods and results of any study are then reviewed by other experts in the field. This process, called peer review, is required before the study is published in a reputable scientific journal. If a treatment proves successful, it is also helpful to follow up with the children on the treatment for longer than the period that was studied to make sure that the beneficial results continue and do not cause any serious long-term side effects.

Which Treatments Have Been Shown to Work?

The treatments for ADHD supported by the strongest evidence are stimulant medications and behavior therapy techniques, often used together. These forms of treatment have been the most studied and validated by the types of rigorous scientific research described previously. For this reason, pediatricians can feel secure in recommending these approaches as proven, safe, and effective, evidence-based, first-line treatments for ADHD.

Many other forms of treatment for ADHD have been tested in studies using the scientific method. Some, such as traditional psychotherapy and cognitive therapy, have been shown through convincing research not to demonstrate positive results in treating the condition's core symptoms. Another group of potential treatments for ADHD has been tested to some extent, but the studies have been too few in number or were conducted with some flaws in study designs, or the results were too ambiguous to prove that the treatment works. Evidence of a treatment's effectiveness may be insufficient if the

- Studies involve too few subjects, so that results cannot be generalized to the ADHD population at large
- "Proof" relies on anecdotal evidence, such as parents' testimonies or one physician's experience with his own patients, rather than on a large group that has been part of a well-designed scientific study
- Study results have not been subjected to the scrutiny of experts who would have reviewed the study prior to publication to identify any possible flaws in the study design or the results

In the following sections, you will find discussions of the evidence supporting or refuting the usefulness of a number of the most popular alternative approaches to treating ADHD and associated problems. Some of these approaches have simply not been studied. Others are based on inaccurate assumptions about the nature of ADHD or its causes, and are therefore unlikely ever to lead to an effective treatment. Still others may eventually be shown to have a significant positive effect, though the current supporting evidence is insufficient, and information about safety is limited. In examining the facts behind the theories, you can not only learn more about these particular treatments, but can also become more comfortable in critically assessing future proposed ADHD treatments on your own.

Your Child's Diet: A Cause and a Cure?

"You are what you eat" is a belief so prevalent in our culture—and true to some extent—that it is easy to understand the temptation to attribute ADHD-type behaviors to some dietary causes, or to believe that particular changes in diet can diminish the symptoms related to the condition. Add to this a widespread concern about the effects of sugar, artificial additives, and other elements in children's diets and it is no wonder that special diets have become the most popular alternative to medication and behavior therapy treatment for ADHD. Recent scientific research has, in fact, supported the belief that eating properly can lower the risk for heart disease and other chronic conditions. Good information on appropriate nutrition is available on the Centers for Disease Control and Prevention Web site at www.cdc.gov/nutrition/everyone/index.html.

Certainly, concerns about nutrition are valid for all children and should not be dismissed. It is also true that some forms of dietary management, and the addition of some trace elements through special supplements, may help with some specific health- or behavior-related problems, and thus are a sensible complementary approach. However, as you will see, none of the special diets designed to treat the symptoms of ADHD have yet been conclusively shown to be effective for most children with the condition. The 2 dietary approaches most discussed for ADHD are supplementing a child's diet by adding nutritional supplements thought to be insufficient or missing, and eliminating one or more foods.

Supplemental Diets

It stands to reason that an adequate diet is necessary for a child's healthy growth. Proper nutrition, including an array of vitamins, minerals, amino acids, and essential fatty acids (EFAs), is particularly necessary in the first few years of life to support brain development and prevent certain neurologic disorders. Even among older children, a lack of certain dietary components, such as protein, or an insufficient number of calories can negatively affect a child's learning and behavioral abilities, and vitamin or mineral deficiencies can certainly interfere with learning over the course of a school year. To date no convincing evidence has shown that a poor diet causes ADHD, or that dietary supplements can be used to successfully treat the condition. Nonetheless, healthy eating and family meals are lifestyle choices generally supported by the American Academy of Pediatrics (AAP).

Megavitamin Therapy

In the 1950s Drs Abram Hoffer and Humphry Osmond began using megavitamins containing large amounts of vitamin B3, vitamin C and, later, pyridoxine (vitamin B6) to treat schizophrenia. This treatment was based on the theory that schizophrenia and some other forms of mental illness are caused by a genetic abnormality that greatly increases the body's vitamin and mineral requirements. By providing patients with enormous doses (megadoses) of these substances, Hoffer and Osmond felt that psychiatrists could provide an "optimum molecular environment for the mind" in which the symptoms of mental illness would diminish or disappear.

In the 1960s the chemist and Nobel Laureate Linus Pauling put his support behind this theory, giving it the name *orthomolecular psychiatry* and greatly increasing its visibility among experts and the general public. In the 1970s Dr Allan Cott claimed that hyperactivity and learning disabilities were also the result of vitamin deficiencies and could be alleviated with megavitamins and large doses of minerals. Treating ADHD symptoms in children with nutritional supplements—supplements that contained at least 10 times the recommended daily allowance of vitamins, minerals, and other necessary elements—became an increasingly popular alternative to stimulant medication, particularly among families who considered megavitamins the more "natural" approach.

Research has failed, however, to reveal significant positive results from megavitamin therapy for children with ADHD. While some early studies resulted in improved classroom attention ratings for subjects taking megavitamins, these studies were marred by the fact that the children, their parents, their teachers, and the researchers were all aware that a given subject was being given this new form of treatment. When the studies were repeated using the double-blind method discussed earlier, so that no one knew whether a particular child was taking a megavitamin or a placebo, no behavioral improvement was shown. In fact, it was discovered that disruptive behavior increased in a significant number of the children given the megavitamins. Studies have also suggested certain abnormalities in the way the liver functions among children on megavitamin therapy, signaling possible toxic effects of this high level of vitamin intake—a strong reminder that "natural" substances are not always safe, especially in the highly "unnatural" doses prescribed here. As a result, experts have concluded that megavitamin therapy for ADHD is of little benefit for nearly all children with the condition—and potentially harmful. In 1976 the AAP Committee on Nutrition issued a formal statement to that effect. No subsequent studies have provided evidence that would change this opinion. This is not to say that children with ADHD should not take any vitamins, just that vitamins at normal doses and even megadoses are not in any way an effective treatment for ADHD.

Other Vitamin and Mineral Supplements

In the wake of the enthusiasm for megavitamin therapy, a number of specific nutritional elements have been studied regarding their possible role in the development of ADHD and their potential for treating the condition. These elements include iron, magnesium, pyridoxine (vitamin B6), and zinc.

All of these substances are known to be necessary for optimal brain development and function. However, no difference between children with or without ADHD has been shown for levels of zinc, iron, magnesium, or vitamin B6, and no links between these low levels and ADHD-type behavior have been established to date. No significant improvement in ADHD behaviors has been demonstrated when supplemental doses of these substances are provided. As with all children, any true nutritional deficiency should be corrected with a standard supplement or a change in daily diet. But supplementation should not exceed the daily recommended allowance because higher levels of some elements (zinc in particular) can prove toxic.

Additional Supplements to Improve Performance

A number of other dietary supplements have been proposed to replace the use of stimulants in treating ADHD. Principal among these are *nootropics, antioxidants,* and *herbs.* Nootropics, specifically a substance called piracetam, have been advocated as cognitive enhancers for children with Down syndrome, dyslexia, and ADHD. While there is no scientific proof of positive effects relating to Down syndrome, one convincing study did show improvement in reading ability and comprehension among children taking piracetam supplements. While there is a rational basis for theorizing that piracetam may also improve ADHD-type behaviors because it is believed to enhance the transmission of the same brain chemicals influenced by stimulant medication (dopamine and noradrenaline), no controlled studies have yet been published, so this treatment cannot be recommended.

Children with ADHD as well as people who eat a modern American diet may have low levels of certain EFAs (including EPA and DHA). In a study of nearly 100 boys, those with lower levels of omega-3 fatty acids had more learning and behavioral problems than boys with normal levels. Studies examining whether omega-3 fatty acids can help improve symptoms of ADHD have found mixed results. A few studies have found that omega-3 fatty acids helped improve behavioral symptoms, but most of these were not well designed. One study that looked at DHA in addition to stimulant therapy found no effect. More research is clearly needed, but for now eating foods that are high in omega-3 fatty acids is certainly a reasonable approach.

Deanol (DMAE), lecithin, and phosphatylserine are other cognitive enhancers (nootropics) frequently found in over-the-counter ADHD remedies available in health food stores or on the Internet. Lecithin and phosphatylserine have not yet been sufficiently studied as treatments for this condition, but DMAE has seemed in one reliable study to be as effective as the stimulant methylphenidate in treating target behaviors. It is clear, then, that though these nootropics cannot currently be recommended as a substitute for stimulants due to insufficient evidence, they are currently being researched and warrant further study as a potential future treatment or complementary supplement for the symptoms of ADHD.

Antioxidants and herbs, used for many centuries in traditional medicine, have only recently come under scientific study. Some of the substances that have been marketed as treatments for ADHD include *pycnogenol,* an antioxidant derived from pine bark; *melatonin,* another antioxidant known to successfully treat sleep cycle disturbances in certain children; *gingko biloba extract,* often used in Europe to treat circulatory and memory disorders; and such herbs as *chamomile, valerian, lemon balm, kava, hops,* and *passion flower.* While melatonin can be useful in addressing sleep disturbances in a child with ADHD, and the herbs mentioned may also be useful as mild sleep aids, the reported positive effects of these antioxidants and herbs as treatments for ADHD core symptoms have been solely anecdotal so far, and there is insufficient scientific evidence to support their use.

If you do decide to administer any of these substances to your child, it is important to inform your child's pediatrician and then carefully monitor their use because some can lead to harmful effects if used in combination with other medications. Gingko biloba extract, for example, must not be taken with aspirin, anticoagulants, or antidepressants, and the herbs listed should not be used when taking sedative medications due to the danger of compounding the sedative's effects. It is necessary to keep in mind that these substances can vary considerably in potency from one preparation to another, and that they are not standardized or regulated by the US Food and Drug Administration.

Elimination Diets

Other theories about the causes of, and treatment for, ADHD have evolved from the hypothesis that certain substances that are *present,* rather than absent, in a child's diet may lead to or worsen the condition. The suspected harmful substances include artificial food additives, preservatives, sugar, or other elements speculated to cause allergic responses or yeast infections that can lead to the development of ADHD. According to these theories, eliminating such elements may eliminate or diminish the symptoms of ADHD.

Feingold Diet

In the mid-1970s a groundswell of concern about the effects of food additives, artificial flavorings, and dyes in the American diet accounted for, in part at least, to the huge popularity of the Feingold Diet as a treatment for ADHD. Dr Benjamin Feingold, a practicing allergist, theorized that these food additives, as well as substances called salicylates (contained in many fruits and vegetables), were causing hyperactivity and learning disabilities in many children. In his book, *Why Your Child Is Hyperactive,* Dr Feingold claimed that when these children were given a special "elimination diet" that omitted these substances, half of them showed a dramatic improvement in behavior. When the elements were reintroduced into the children's diet, the symptoms returned. Most controlled studies do not support that elimination of these substances leads to better outcome for children with ADHD. Only about 2% of children with ADHD on the Feingold diet have shown consistent behavioral improvement when these food dyes were eliminated. However, reduction of processed foods that contain artificial dyes and substitution of healthy foods may in general promote better long-term health. Moreover, the behavior management strategies that parents must use to change a child's eating behavior from frequent use of candies and processed foods to healthy choices are the same techniques that are used to improve concentration and increase work production.

Diets Eliminating Sensitizing Food Substances

In the decades since the Feingold Diet was introduced, studies of the impact of diet on behavioral disorders have become more sophisticated and reliable. Newer research has shown that behavioral improvement using elimination diets is more likely in children who have inhaled and food allergies, a family history of migraines, and food reactivity. Younger children seem to be the most responsive. Whole foods like milk, nuts, wheat, fish, and soy have been implicated in addition to additives. Elimination diets can sometimes influence sleep and mood disturbances as well as ADHD symptoms. Sensitivities to substances in the environment—in medicines, clothes, water, our homes, the air, and so on—have also been studied as they relate to children's health and behavior. The results have shown a link between sensitizing foods and some health and behavior problems in a small percentage of children with ADHD. In most cases, these children experience a variety of coexisting health and behavioral difficulties in addition to ADHD—particularly sleep-related and neurologic problems. They are also likely to have a family history of food sensitivities or migraine headaches.

Because this link has been established, if food or additive sensitivities are highly suspected in your child, he may be tested for them by first eliminating an entire range of common foods (typically milk, soy, wheat, corn, citrus, and peanuts) for 2 to 4 weeks. If his symptoms improve—signaling the possible presence of a food sensitivity—the range of foods can be restored to his diet, then one food at a time can be removed for a short period, with the results being monitored. This process can continue until the correct substance has been identified or all likely possibilities have been exhausted. This procedure may be difficult to carry out, and it is advised that if you are interested you should do this along with a physician or certified dietician. It is extremely important to pick countable targets (such as "2 or fewer tantrums per day") rather than general impressions ("will demonstrate better behavior").

Meanwhile, it is important to understand that for most children with ADHD who do not have food sensitivities (and for some who do), elimination diets are not effective treatments for ADHD itself. If your child is on a special diet, you will need to make sure it is not replacing a more effective treatment for ADHD symptoms. In most cases, stimulant medication, behavior therapy, and the other measures described in previous chapters will have a much clearer positive effect on your child's ADHD-related behaviors, while a well-balanced diet with few processed foods may improve his general health and attitude.

Sugar-Free Diets

Humans are naturally attracted to sugar because it tastes good and because our bodies rely on glucose—the form of sugar found in natural foods—for metabolic processes. Like many other children, children with ADHD often have strong sugar cravings, and this has contributed to the belief that sugar and candy consumption can cause hyperactive behavior. A great deal of objective evidence, however, has shown that this assumption is untrue for most children with or without ADHD. While one early study did reveal a link between high sugar consumption and hyperactive behavior, there was no evidence that one caused the other or that the behavior problems were not due to different parenting styles or other factors. A number of subsequent scientifically rigorous studies could not demonstrate any adverse effects of sugar on the behavior of children. As for children with ADHD, sugar consumption has not been shown to cause or enhance ADHD-related behavior.

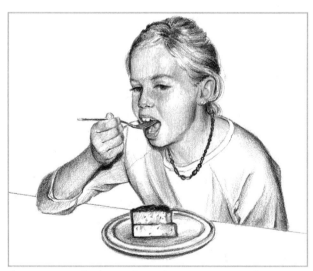

Sugar consumption has not been shown to cause or enhance ADHD-related behavior. Of course, allowing sugar only in moderation makes sense for any child.

Of course, allowing sugar only in moderation makes sense for any child. Again, assuming leadership within the family, making healthy choices about what is offered to the child, and using behavior management to educate children to reduce sugar and processed food may have general benefits. If your child shows an uncontrollable craving for sugar and carbohydrates, discuss this with his pediatrician. Aside from issues relating to general health, a sugar-free diet is not considered a useful tool in treating ADHD. Researchers have found again and again that the simple elimination of sugar or candy, with few exceptions, does not help children with ADHD.

Aspartame-Free Diet

Aspartame, an artificial sweetener that became available in the early 1980s, consists of amino acids that cross from the bloodstream into the brain to affect brain function. (Interestingly, it was used as the placebo in some of the studies of sugar's effects on behavior.) It was believed that among individuals susceptible to this substance, aspartame might lead to seizures or ADHD-type behaviors. No such effects have been demonstrated, however, and elimination of aspartame for children with ADHD is not considered an effective treatment except for children with phenylketonuria, a chemical disorder that prevents some people from being able to break down or metabolize aspartame.

Yeast- or Fungus-Free Diets

In the mid-1980s, Dr William Crook, a practicing pediatrician and allergist, popularized the theory that hyperactivity, irritability, and learning disorders in children could be caused by chronic candida (yeast) infection. The theory behind this is that when the immune system is weakened, or when antibiotics are being taken, "friendly" bacteria in the gastrointestinal system are eliminated and yeast can take over. Those who feel that this process has a deleterious role in children with ADHD believe that toxins produced by a yeast overgrowth weaken the immune system and make an individual susceptible to ADHD. Because of this they support the use of antifungal agents and sugar restriction. There are no sound studies that support this hypothesis or this treatment.

Vision, Inner-Ear, Auditory Integration, and Sensory Integration Problems

An entire class of theories about the causes of ADHD and effective treatments for it centers on the workings of the senses. Problems relating to sight, hearing, balance controlled by the inner ear, sensory integration, and so on have been proposed as underlying conditions that lead to ADHD and accompanying problems and disorders. Each theory is linked to a treatment approach, and each form of treatment is supported by a large number of vocal enthusiasts. The theory behind sensory integration therapy, done by occupational therapists, is that through structured and constant movement, a child's brain can learn to integrate and better react to sensory messages. There is as yet no evidence that it helps children with ADHD. One of the tools that evidence-based medicine has available is that of meta-analysis. Meta-analysis searches out all studies that have been done with rigorous methods, such as including placebos, following children as the study is proceeding (prospective), and where neither the investigator or the parents know if the treatment their child is receiving is the study treatment or the placebo (double-blind). Meta-analyses studies of several disabling conditions have not found sensory integration to be significantly helpful. These studies did not include children with ADHD, and there is no evidence-based support at this time for its use with children who have been diagnosed with ADHD.

Optometric Training

Optometric training, a kind of eye training for children with learning disabilities, is based on the theory that faulty eye movements and problems in visual perception can cause dyslexia, language disorders, and other learning problems that frequently accompany ADHD. Named behavioral optometry by the optometrists who developed and support this form of therapy, the treatment consists of teaching children specific visual skills as a way of improving learning. These skills include tracking moving objects, fixating on or locating objects quickly and accurately, encouraging both eyes to work together successfully, and changing focus efficiently. The skills are taught through the use of eye exercises and special colored or prismatic lenses. Optometric training is often supplemented with training in academic skills, nutrition, and personal relationships. This treatment is frequently quite expensive.

Little research has supported the theory that dyslexia or other learning disabilities are caused by vision defects or problems, and thus vision training is an ineffective approach to reading and learning disabilities. In 1984 the AAP, along with the American Association for Pediatric Ophthalmology and Strabismus and the American Academy of Ophthalmology, issued a policy statement affirming that no known scientific evidence "supports the claims for improving the academic abilities of dyslexic or learning-disabled children with treatment based on visual training, including muscle exercises, ocular pursuit or tracking exercises, or glasses (with or without bifocals or prisms)."

Because vision training is not only ineffective but may delay more effective treatment for coexisting learning disabilities, it is not recommended. There have been no studies on optometric training for children with ADHD, despite its widespread use.

Interactive Metronome

Difficulties with auditory integration—that is, organizing, attending to, and making sense out of information while listening—have also been suspected as a cause of ADHD. One recent approach has been to use interactive metronome training. The interactive metronome is a computerized version of the metronomes used by musicians to help train them to keep time at a constant rate. It produces a rhythmic beat that users attempt to match by tapping their hand or foot. The program gives children feedback on their accuracy. The theory behind this is that children will gain motor planning and timing skills. These skills have been found suboptimal in many children with ADHD. Incoordination is a frequent accompaniment to ADHD because children with ADHD often act motorically before thinking (they are impulsive). Fine motor skills are sometimes helped considerably with stimulant medication. There is one well-done study showing benefits from interactive metronome in boys with ADHD for a wide range of activities, but additional research would need to be done before this treatment could be generally recommended for children with ADHD.

Neurofeedback, Hypnotherapy, and Guided Imagery

A number of proposed treatments for ADHD—including hypnotherapy, self-hypnosis, guided imagery, neurofeedback, and relaxation training—are aimed at helping a child begin to regulate his own behavior and psychological state. The fact that these techniques can be used quite successfully for children in other areas of self-regulation (headache management, teaching bowel control, etc) increases their appeal as a form of treatment.

Hypnotherapy has not been shown to significantly improve the core symptoms of ADHD, though it may improve such accompanying problems as sleep problems and tics when used as part of an integrated treatment approach. One difference between the use of hypnotherapy for headaches versus ADHD is that children learn to institute the self-hypnosis at the early signs of a headache. There is no comparable "trigger" with ADHD, and children cannot do self-hypnosis all day long.

Neurofeedback treatment involves placing electrodes on a child's head to monitor brain activity. Children are asked, for example, to change the aspects of a video game (for example "making the sun set with your mind"), which happens when their brainwaves are of a desired frequency. The theory is that learning to do this increases their arousal levels, improves their attention, and results in reductions in hyperactive-impulsive behaviors. This is based on findings that many children with ADHD show low levels of arousal in frontal brain areas, with excess of theta (daydreamy) waves and deficit of beta waves (indicators of a highly focused mind), thereby reducing ADHD. The studies on the use of neurofeedback to date have been criticized for lacking the appropriate controls or the random assignment of test subjects to the treatment or sham treatment groups. It should also be pointed out that neurofeedback treatment is an expensive approach to treating ADHD.

Homeopathy

Homeopathy, a therapeutic approach developed in the 1800s that is especially popular in Europe, springs from the concept that illness results from a disorder of "vital energies," and that these energies must be restored if a patient is to recover. Vital energies can be restored through the use of diluted animal, plant, or mineral extracts designed to treat specific symptoms. These treatments have been shown to be more effective than placebos in reliable scientific studies, though the reason for this is not yet known. Homeopathic treatment for ADHD, increasingly widespread in the United States as individual accounts of success have spread, has been demonstrated effective in one initial study in improving ADHD-type behavior, although the study failed to use a fully double-blind design. Though the mechanisms underlying this treatment are still not scientifically defined, the success of the study merits further investigation of homeopathy as a treatment for ADHD, but it cannot be recommended as a proven therapy at this time. If you do become interested in using this approach, be sure to discuss your plans first with your child's physician. Some extracts can interact negatively with medications your child may be taking.

Chiropractic

Chiropractic is a medical system based on the theory that disease and disorders are caused by a misalignment of the bones, especially in the spine, that obstructs proper nerve functions, and that adjustments and spinal manipulations can restore health. Some chiropractors believe that ADHD can be treated with spinal adjustments as well as sensory stimulation, including various frequencies of light and sound. Others believe that realigning the sphenoid bone at the base of the skull and the temporal bones on the side of the head can address the symptoms of ADHD and learning disabilities. The theory is that when these bones are malaligned, an unequal pressure is created in different brain areas. These treatments are not compatible with present views of the causes of ADHD and learning disorders, and there is no information on the effectiveness of these approaches.

Using The Internet

An excellent source of medical information and valuable advice, the Internet can also be the source of a great deal of dubious health-related theories, "facts," and testimonials. In searching the Internet for information about a proposed ADHD treatment—or for any other information about ADHD and related conditions—it is always a good idea to start with the most reliable general information Web sites and expand from there. The Web sites listed in the Resources section on page 311 are excellent first steps. They can provide you with links to more specific information, support groups, and sources of government information.

A good way to quickly ascertain the reliability of an Internet resource is to look at the suffix of its Web site address. Government information Web site addresses end in ".gov." These include sites such as the National Institutes of Health and National Institute of Mental Health and have a wealth of health-related teaching materials for the general public. Nonprofit organizations, such as the AAP and the advocacy organization Children and Adults with Attention-Deficit/Hyperactivity Disorder (CHADD), have Web sites ending in ".org"—however, not all organizations put out materials as reliable as the materials from these 2 organizations. Academic Web sites have ".edu" suffixes on their Internet addresses, and many of these have evidence-based educational materials geared toward parents. Web sites with the suffixes ".com" generally are commercial Web sites not necessarily affiliated with an educational entity or a source of reliable information.

Take some time to look at these sites—and be sure to explore any Web site first before having your child follow its recommendations.

New Remedies for ADHD: You Be the Judge

Claims about a new treatment can be difficult to resist. Who wouldn't love to find a "miraculous" new treatment that would completely eradicate the symptoms of ADHD and involve only healthy, "natural" substances that appear in our ordinary diet? Yet the very terms that tap into your longing to use them to conquer this condition—terms such as *cutting-edge, amazing,* and *revolutionary*—should also serve as signals that it is time to take a hard look at the evidence that backs such claims up. Many of the proponents of these cures carry impressive initials after their names—many are "doctors" or "professors" of some kind. Many are sincere in their belief that they have found a major treatment or even a cure for this complex and often baffling disorder. Yet sincerity—even passionate belief—is not enough to render a treatment effective.

In reviewing the summaries of the popular ADHD-related theories and treatments described previously, you have seen how important it is to go beyond proponents' claims—no matter how convincing or intuitively "right" they may seem—to examine the scientific research backing up those assertions. As you encounter news of new proposed treatments for ADHD, ask yourself the questions below, provided by CHADD. (See fact sheets at www.chadd.org.)

Will it work for my child?

Suspect an unproven remedy if it

- Claims it will work for everyone with ADHD and other health problems
- Uses only case histories or testimonials as proof
- Cites only one study as proof
- Cites a study without a control (comparison) group

How safe is it?

Suspect an unproven remedy if it

- Comes without directions for proper use
- Does not list contents
- Has no information or warnings about side effects
- Is described as harmless or natural (Remember, most medication is developed from natural sources, but "natural" treatments may still be ineffective or harmful.)

How is it promoted?

Suspect an unproven remedy if it

- Claims it is based on a secret formula
- Claims that it will work immediately and permanently for everyone with ADHD
- Is described as "astonishing," "miraculous," or an "amazing breakthrough"
- Claims it cures ADHD
- Is available from only one source
- Is promoted only through infomercials, self-promoting books, or by mail order
- Claims that treatment is being suppressed or unfairly attacked by the medical establishment

Even when an alternative treatment has been shown to be potentially useful for specific symptoms or behaviors that have been targeted for your child, it is important to consider, and to discuss with your child's pediatrician, whether it is more effective than already proven treatments, whether it may involve any uncomfortable or dangerous side effects or health hazards, how expensive it is, and how difficult it is for your family to implement. If your child's pediatrician is not knowledgeable about the approach in question, you will need to do much of the research yourself through the avenues discussed previously.

Keep in mind that the first and most important step in choosing the best treatment for your child is obtaining a full and accurate diagnosis of his ADHD and any coexisting problems or conditions. A standard medical evaluation is also necessary to learn whether your child could benefit from special treatment for any nutritional, vision, hearing, or other problem. Standard treatments, such as stimulant medication and behavioral therapy, should always be considered as first-line approaches for ADHD. If you, your child, and his treatment team prefer an alternative treatment, the scientific validity of the treatment and its appropriateness for your child needs to be carefully reviewed, analyzed, and discussed.

Pediatricians, like parents, have many different views of the role of complementary and alternative treatments in the treatment of children diagnosed with ADHD. Physicians can play a constructive role in helping families make these kinds of treatment choices by reviewing the stated goals or effects claimed for a given treatment, the state of evidence to support or discourage use of the treatment, and a review of known or potential side effects. As you've seen from the material in this chapter, there are many categories of complementary and alternative treatments: those that have been found to be effective, those that have not been proven to be effective, those that have been shown to be ineffective, and those that can have dangerous effects or side effects. Common sense would lead to the approach of considering the use of proven treatments as the foundation of a sound plan, and then to consider treatments that are unproven, while avoiding treatments that can be dangerous. Parents may find themselves using treatments that have been shown to be ineffective from time to time, and feel that they might be working, but remain unsure. If you choose to use some of these complementary treatments it can be very helpful to introduce only one new treatment at a time in a systematic way. One suggestion for introducing the treatment is to make a list of changes that you hope to see if the treatment is effective before you start it. Make the items on your list countable (as suggested in other parts of this book)—for example, "James will go from 40% (his present baseline) missing assignments per week to 25%." Also commit to the time frame in which you expect to see the change. For supplements and dietary manipulations you should be able to see differences within a month or two. For expensive treatments you may need to specify the funds you are willing to commit and then calculate the time frame based on that funding. After the designated amount of time, if these goals are achieved, stop the treatment and see if the number of missing assignments returns to the baseline number. If the problem reoccurs start the treatment again and see if it improves again. Make sure that your own behavior remains neutral in this personal experiment so that your expectations do not alter the outcomes. Many of these complementary and alternative treatments can add structure, commitment, and hope to families' lives even if they are not totally healing.

Chapter 11

ADHD in Adolescence

For every child, with or without attention-deficit/hyperactivity disorder (ADHD), adolescence is a time of profound change—a time of transitioning from full dependence on and identification with his family toward a separate, independent adult self. Although it was previously believed that most children outgrow ADHD by their teenage years, and that the condition rarely continues into adulthood, recent research has shown that ADHD persists into adolescence and beyond for at least 65% of children diagnosed with the condition. As the parent of a teenager with ADHD, you will need to understand and prepare for the many ways in which this normal developmental process can affect your child's academic (school) and social performance and his relationship with you—as well as how ADHD may affect his overall development. In some cases, ADHD symptoms tend to become subtler during the teenage years, although even in these adolescents it can often be quite valuable to continue treatment. (Treatment plans will need to be reviewed carefully and regularly.)

Adolescence may seem to bring on a wider gap between teenagers and their peers. Some recent studies have shown a significant lag in brain maturity, particularly in the prefrontal cortex—the area that is responsible for paying attention, planning motor activities like writing; impulse control; and the systems that temporarily store and manage the information required to carry out complex tasks such as learning, reasoning, and comprehension (working memory). This needs to be considered while, at the same time, you respect your teenager's need to become progressively independent. You may also need to reconsider your teenager's medication plan, for example, as his activities expand. His willingness to take medication may waver as he resists seeming "different" from his peers. The increasing demands of middle school and high school may require more attention to planning and staying organized or to changes in his educational plan. At home your teenager may respond negatively to parenting techniques you once found effective—and insist on approving any new approaches you want to use. Meanwhile the presence of ADHD may be accompanied by delays in the development of skills necessary to support an increasingly independent life.

Having said all this, remember that your child is a teenager first and foremost, and don't over-think what part of his behavior is from "being a teenager" and what part is connected to ADHD. Many parents worry way too much and this gets in the way of their relationship with their teens and pushes their teens away from them. All the teens may hear is "gloom and doom." Teenagers are growing and developing daily, weekly, monthly, in small and often imperceptible ways. Almost all will be responsible adults. Like other parents of adolescents, offer support, deal with the challenges along the way, provide love and praise, and wait while watching the process of maturation unfold. Also consider that people with ADHD have to work hard, probably harder than those without it. Successful teenagers with ADHD need to understand this to succeed. This may be easier, if as children they have learned that challenges can be viewed as obstacles to overcome, rather than debilitating things that happen "to them" that they are powerless to change.

Clearly, adolescence is a challenging time for your entire family. However, it is also a time of great promise as your teenager begins to explore his potential as a unique human being with a great deal to offer the world. Finding the ideal balance between protection and empowerment will be a difficult task for you as a parent, yet there is nothing more exciting than watching your teenager start to fully accept, manage, and master his own situation. Your earlier efforts to help your child take control of his own progress will start to pay off now as he enters early adulthood.

This chapter will outline the additional steps necessary to

- Help your teenager meet new academic challenges.
- Help him manage new social and emotional pressures.
- Help you parent more effectively.
- Learn to take care of yourself as he works on becoming more independent.

ADHD and Your Teenager's Development

Every teenager's primary developmental task is to begin the process of "individuation," or the creation of a sense of self separate from his identity with his family. A child's sense of his own uniqueness begins early in life, of course, but kicks into high gear at around age 11 or 12 years. One early step in this individuation process—a step that will occupy much of your child's energy for the next few years—is to establish as clearly as possible the ways in which he is not like you. Once he feels that these differences or boundaries have been securely defined, he can move in later adolescence toward understanding who he is.

Establishing a separate sense of self is not easy for the younger teenager. Even he may not always understand why he so frequently tunes you out, slams his bedroom door when he is angry, or hides his journal—and his own behavior may confuse or upset him at times. His personal identity can be so fragile that even a minor threat, such as a parent's criticism or a sibling's teasing, may lead to extremely defensive behavior. At the same time, his developing sense of who he is can leave him vulnerable to peer pressure and other potentially negative outside influences. Even with his ADHD-related behavior, he needs to be reminded that he is not "bad" or "stupid," but rather that he needs help in certain areas, just as a teenager with asthma or other medical conditions needs to take steps to eliminate major roadblocks to his functioning.

While your teenager continues to mature, the typical adolescent's developmental tasks—his need to separate from his parents, define himself, fit in with his peers—put him at greater risk than in earlier childhood for academic failure; experimentation with tobacco, drugs, or alcohol; early sexual activity; and all of the other types of activity that keep parents up at night. Most teenagers develop new strengths during these years that help them with decision-making on their own as their parents' influence starts to fade. They improve their ability to think long term, resist momentary impulses, and regulate their own behavior. Teenagers with ADHD, however, often lag behind in these areas, while experiencing the same need for independence as their peers. At the same time, certain ADHD-related behaviors may actually increase the risk that your child will engage in some of the self-defeating activities that many other teenagers may avoid. In part, this is because teenagers with ADHD can lack varied degrees of insight into their own functioning and may be less able to realistically assess their abilities than their peers. This makes self-management more difficult, and creates a key paradox because it occurs at exactly the time that they need to assume greater control of their lives.

The manner in which ADHD is manifested during adolescence depends on its severity, sub-type (predominantly hyperactive-impulsive–, inattentive-, or combined-type ADHD), and your teenager's particular profile of strengths and weaknesses. His ADHD-related behavior is also strongly affected by his stage of development; his risk-taking behaviors; and the presence of any coexisting conditions, such as depression, learning disabilities, or anxiety disorder. The quality of his home and school environment can also make an enormous difference in how well he functions in his daily life. As a result, teenagers with ADHD tend to behave in widely varying ways. A teenager with hyperactive-impulsive ADHD and a coexisting disruptive behavior disorder may get into fights constantly at school and be suspended several times each semester, while another with inattentive-type ADHD and depression may fall behind in school, lose self-esteem, and escape special notice until he starts "self-medicating" with marijuana or alcohol. A teenager with good verbal and language skills may have managed to keep up his grades and go undiagnosed for ADHD in elementary and middle school, but may start to fail his high school courses as the demands for a high level of work production expose his organizational weaknesses. Another teenager who has participated in his ADHD treatment all along and experienced successes may show marked improvement at school and with friends as he grows able to help manage his own medication and take greater control of his areas of strength and weakness. Some studies have shown differences in concerns between teenage boys and girls. Compared with other girls, some girls with ADHD are more likely to experience more depression, anxiety, distress, poor teacher relationships, stress, feelings that they cannot control their own fate, and more struggles with academics. Compared with boys with ADHD, girls with ADHD report more anxiety, distress, and difficulty taking charge of their own problems.

Each subtype of ADHD can present its own challenges during adolescence. By educating yourself about these issues and how they come into play in different ways for different teenagers, you can better support your child as he proceeds through this new developmental stage.

Poor Impulse Control

Most adolescents act impulsively now and then, and teenagers are known for favoring short-term pleasures over long-term benefits. Teenagers with hyperactive-impulsive– or combined-type ADHD, however, can have much more difficulty than others in regulating their impulses, even when they know their behavior is self-destructive. As when he was younger, your child may still act first and think later—but now the stakes are higher and impulsiveness can potentially lead to substance abuse, aggressive behavior, unprotected sex, reckless driving, or other high-risk situations. Even minor impulsive behavior—interrupting others, fidgeting at his desk—may cause academic or social problems for your teenager as others expect more "mature" behavior despite the presence of ADHD.

IS IT ADOLESCENCE OR ADHD?

When faced with a disruptive 14-year-old, a 10th-grader with a sudden drop in grades, or a high school junior who regularly ignores the curfews you impose, it can be difficult if not impossible to tell whether such behavior is part of normal adolescent development or an aspect of your child's ADHD. As was the case earlier in childhood, behaviors related to ADHD resemble those of teenagers without ADHD, but can be at the more extreme end of the continuum and are likely to continue for months or years after they have diminished in individuals without ADHD.

In the end, it is not really important to know whether a particular behavior is or is not ADHD-related because your response in either case should be the same. Unacceptable behaviors need to be met with consistent limits and appropriate consequences. Your teenager's potentially greater difficulties with impulse control, focusing, and organizing and long-term planning may require extra consistency, structure, and thought on your part—but he would benefit from these measures even if he does not have ADHD.

It is important for you and your teenager to understand that behaving impulsively is not a moral failure on his part, but an aspect of his ADHD that requires special attention during this period. Your adolescent will benefit from learning about ways to minimize the potentially damaging effects of this behavior. Later in this chapter, you will find a number of suggestions that may help with managing impulsiveness in your teenager's personal, academic, and social life.

Difficulty Focusing and Organizing

Teenagers with predominantly inattentive- or combined-type ADHD generally do not concentrate or sustain their attention as well as their classmates. At times they can find it almost impossible to focus on a class lecture, take good notes, or complete homework or other tasks. Others may characterize them as "flighty" or "daydreamy," but these behaviors are aspects of ADHD, not willful behaviors or personality traits. Clearly, such difficulties can get in the way of your teenager's desire to take greater control of his own academic success. He may start the school year determined to bring home a "great" report card, and have no idea why he is struggling with his grades so much more than his peers. An inability to focus can also defeat his efforts to succeed socially or at a job. Help your teenager understand that extra support may be necessary to help him achieve the higher demands of adolescence, and that this temporary support is a necessary step along the road toward independence.

Problems With Long-term Planning

The adolescent surge toward independence is accompanied by a burst of maturation that helps most teenagers achieve their eventual goal of successful individuation. This development centers on what are called executive functions—the ability to plan ahead, conceptualize, and prioritize the steps necessary to reach a goal, and move systematically and non-impulsively toward that goal until it has been achieved. Teenagers with ADHD, however, can lag behind in this form of maturation. As a result, while your teenager may be as determined as his peers to "control his own destiny"—wanting to get a job or apply to colleges all on his own—he may often need extra support in achieving these goals. Discuss ahead of time how you and others can help and support him to take the steps he needs to succeed. Help him understand that a key to being a truly self-sufficient person includes knowing when and how to seek assistance—whether that involves scheduling a meeting with his teacher, asking a counselor for special guidance, or using a coach to help him organize and plan his homework.

Low Self-esteem

Teenagers with ADHD can experience a good deal of difficulty in academic, social, or personal areas. Even with your support and empathy, such experiences can decrease your child's confidence and self-esteem. Low self-esteem may lead him to refuse medication, avoid special educational activities, or do anything else that might make him appear or

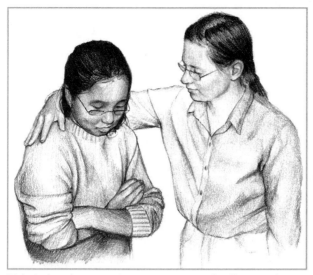

Make it clear that you support your teenager. It will mean a lot to your teenager to know that you will always be in her corner.

feel different from his peers. Lack of confidence may also leave teenagers with ADHD more vulnerable to peer pressure regarding drug use or other dangerous behaviors as they try to prove they are as "cool" as anyone else. This is an age when children need to be able to follow their passions and identify islands of competence. It is important to support these passions, even if they are activities like video games, and to consider that these activities can model that learning skills through repetition and hard work pay off. This can help teenagers see that they are competent and can learn anything by applying the same persistence to school or music or whatever.

Independence Issues

Teenagers want and expect to attend parties, get a driver's license, and generally enjoy increasing amounts of privacy and independence with each passing year. Yet it is important for you and your teenager to understand that having ADHD can potentially make some activities more risky, and these may need to be monitored more closely than for his peers without ADHD. A teenager dealing with inattention, for example, may need to agree to drive only while his stimulant medication is in effect. If your child's problems completing homework have led to poor or failing grades, he may need help with reviewing his work each night to be sure he has met his goals. Of course, your teenager is likely to resent and resist some of these potentially helpful measures, but he will also rely on you to set and enforce necessary limits. You can make it easier for him to accept this continued dependence by problem-solving with him in a way that respects his needs by making sure that he is invited to help create the rules and routines he needs.

Your Teenager's Treatment Plan

The best strategy for preparing your child to successfully manage the challenges that ADHD imposes during adolescence is to have encouraged him to be actively engaged in all elements of his treatment plan in his preteen years.

A PARENT'S STORY

Feeling Involved

"We've always made it a point to have Seth be part of his school conferences and medical visits. When he was in grade school he dreaded his visits to his pediatrician to discuss his treatment. He would tell us, 'She always asks me the same questions about school and about my medicine, and always tells me the same things about how my medicine works.' Then when he was about 11 she started meeting with him alone for part of our visits, and he would usually come out with a list of three or four things that he was going to work on. Eventually we began to notice that Seth was beginning to take more responsibility on his own for making sure that his homework got into his backpack before he left for school, and he would remind us if we forgot to put out his medication in the morning. By the time he was in eleventh grade he had pretty much taken over the responsibility for his medication and even asked us if we could get him a coach/tutor to help him organize one of his long-term projects. We feel like we did something right by keeping him involved in his own treatment."

Joyce, Chicago, IL

PREDICTORS OF SUCCESS DURING ADOLESCENCE

Some of the most important factors in teenagers with ADHD who do the best during adolescence include

- Early intervention
- Self-understanding and acceptance of problems and issues
- A supportive family
- An understanding and developmentally attuned school system
- An appropriate Individualized Education Program (IEP) if indicated
- A willingness to engage in appropriate counseling, mentoring relationships, and "coaching" surrounding production and completion of work

PREDICTORS OF SUCCESS DURING ADOLESCENCE (CONTINUED)

Some of the highest-risk factors leading to negative outcomes for teenagers with ADHD include

- Delayed intervention/treatment
- An ongoing cycle of failure
- Serious behavior problems in school
- Significant substance abuse
- Medication refusal
- Damaged self-esteem resulting from problems being viewed as character flaws rather than ADHD-related behaviors
- Giving up or lack of "motivation"

Changing Treatment Needs

Throughout this book, you have been encouraged to continue addressing your child's functioning problems and to meet regularly with his treatment team to reassess his needs. Regular review sessions may become especially important as your child enters adolescence and academic, social, and emotional pressures start to increase. As the parent of a teenager with ADHD, it will be important to have an agreed-on system to keep track of homework production and grades, but also to arrange with teachers for regular, brief meetings or telephone conferences about progress. Weekly home-school report cards and other monitoring tools (see Chapter 7) used with younger teenagers can help reveal any academic or behavioral problems before they cause too much damage, and lead to helpful changes in treatment or education programs. Chances are your teenager may object at some point to this level of scrutiny, which is more than his peers without ADHD probably receive. To counterbalance this, make sure that you provide ample opportunities for him to assert his autonomy in as many appropriate situations as possible, and allow him to direct as much of the monitoring system as is developmentally appropriate.

Aside from changing academic needs, your teenager may experience greater social conflict and increased emotional stress during middle school and high school. You may hear about some of these problems—particularly disruptive behavioral issues—from school personnel. Other important changes—increases in depression or anxiety, increasing social rejection, plunging self-esteem—may remain virtually invisible to you as a parent. As your child begins the normal adolescent process of separating from you described previously, he is less likely to confide in you about these types of problems. For this reason, it is very important to allow time for him to meet privately with his doctor during every treatment review session to ensure that he receives a careful screening for these symptoms and additional diagnostic work or help if indicated.

Keep in mind that the older your child gets, the more aware he is of the special attention he is receiving, and the more sensitive he will be to what this says about who he is and what his capabilities are. The more you can present monitoring techniques as proactive tools for his own self-empowerment, rather than limits to his personal growth, the more positive his attitude toward his treatment is likely to be.

Medication Management

If your child has been successfully treated with medication in the past, your medication management plan should be carefully reviewed as adolescence begins. There is no hard-and-fast rule about the changing medication needs of teenagers. It used to be thought that children "outgrow" ADHD sometime in their teenage years, and medication was often stopped at that time. We now know that although hyperactivity often becomes less of a problem, impulsive behavior and inattention usually persist. The commonly used stimulant medications have been found to provide benefits for most teenagers with ADHD, and are effective in both teenage boys and girls.

Teenagers do not necessarily need changes in their medication dosage even after the large growth spurts that adolescence brings. Your teenager's dose, however, may need to be increased or lowered on the basis of his ability to function well academically, behaviorally, and socially. Medication dosing needs sometimes change because of increased homework demands, or complex schedules. If your teenager leaves for school at 7:30 in the morning, has soccer practice after school, and does not get to his homework until 8:00 pm, even a 12-hour preparation of stimulant medication may have worn off by that time. Some teenagers solve this by going back to an 8-hour preparation for the school day, and then synchronizing a shorter-acting (4-hour) dose to cover their homework time.

Your teenager craves independence, yet the presence of ADHD means he will probably need extra structure and support from you. At times, he may resist taking his ADHD medication and he may argue about following your and your doctor's guidelines for managing medication. Be honest with him about your concerns, and ask for his help in designing a medication routine that will best address his needs as well as your concerns. You might agree, for example, that he will be responsible for remembering to take his medication, unless more than 10% of his pills remain untaken on a weekly pill count. If conflicts arise over the balance between limits and personal freedom, ask your teenager's pediatrician, psychologist, or school counselor to help mediate or contribute ideas. Some teenagers dislike taking medication, stating that they don't feel "themselves." This can be viewed the same as a side effect and you may need to work to try to adjust the dose of medication to minimize that. This gives teenagers power and input into their medication. When they refuse to take medication or want a trial off medication this should be viewed as a positive, and taken seriously. If your teenager feels that he can succeed without medication, encourage him to set up an alternative plan that works. Going back on medication may become the default option. Remember, you don't *want* them to take medications; you want them to succeed whether it's on or off medication.

So if your teenager continues to question the effectiveness of stimulant medication, or states a desire to discontinue medication altogether, his pediatrician might help him set up a carefully monitored "trial" on and off medication that will include careful teacher observations of relevant academic, behavioral, or social concerns for a specified period. The teacher will make these observations without knowing which period is off and which is on. Your son can also keep a careful diary of his own observations. The observations can be reviewed after the trial for any significant differences in homework completion, grades, etc, on and off medication, and then make a better informed decision about whether to continue medication as a part of his treatment plan. Conducting such a trial will also respect your child's need to participate in decision-making about treatment. This type of activity can be particularly effective for skeptical teenagers who prefer to "see" before they "believe." Medical professionals can also provide your teenager with books and videotapes about ADHD treatment, and put him in touch with ADHD support groups that can help him understand how others have learned to manage their ADHD. Remaining on medication is not an easy choice for teenagers.

A TEENAGER'S STORY

Feelings About Medication

A high school student recently wrote, "I don't want to take my medication because I don't like the way it makes feel and it makes me lose weight, which hurts me in football. My friends and family have their own advice for me. My good friend Dylan said I should stay on the medication. He thinks that I am more relaxed and that I am more focused on topics when I'm taking medication. My other friend Jacob thinks that I should stop taking the medication. In his opinion I am more of a loner when I am on the medication and I avoid people. It's true. I liked it better when we used to hang out more. My mom thinks that the medication is great for me. She feels that I am more organized with my homework in school and that I write a lot neater. She also noticed that I memorize faster and that she doesn't need to study with me as much. Since I started taking medication, I have proved anyone who thought I was stupid wrong. Now my mom is helping me pick out a college to attend. I am sure that I would slip up if I did not take my pills and then lose my chance at college."

Adapted wih permission from: Heimerl J. *ADD drugs? not easy to take.* Twin Cities Daily Planet. November 30, 2009. Copyright © Three Sixty Journalism.

STICKING TO A MEDICATION SCHEDULE

Teenagers who are more likely to adhere to the prescribed use of stimulant medications are more likely to have

- A positive self-concept
- Family stability
- Confidence in their ability to solve problems
- Simplified medication schedules
- The absence of side effects from medications
- A positive relationship with their doctor

Adapted with permission from Reiff MI. Case report: An adolescent who no longer wants to take medication. *Consultant for Pediatricians.* August 2007;(suppl):12.

Abuse of Stimulant Medication

For a minority of teenagers with ADHD, resistance to taking stimulant medication may be less of a problem than overuse. Stimulants are classified as Schedule II drugs by the US Drug Enforcement Administration and, sooner or later, teenagers who take stimulant medication usually become aware of its "street value." Your child may be tempted at some point to give or sell his medication to others, or to take more than the prescribed dose himself. While it is a fact of life that most teenagers experiment with some form of high-risk behavior, such as a single episode of alcohol or drug experimentation, the presence of ADHD makes it especially important for you (and, ideally, your child's pediatrician) to discuss the dangers of drug abuse with him and to monitor his medication use. Teenagers who are doing well on a treatment plan that may include taking stimulant medications are generally less likely to abuse stimulants than those who do not have a treatment plan in place and are not taking medication, and because of this are experiencing low self-esteem, are more impulsive, and are more inclined to take risks. If your child has a coexisting behavioral disorder, or has abused or sold medication in the past, develop a system for dispensing medication that prevents these possibilities to the greatest extent possible.

Meeting New Academic Challenges

It is easy to understand how a teenager with these types of difficulties could quickly become overwhelmed by the increasing academic demands of middle school and high school. While some students with ADHD—particularly those with milder symptoms, good parental support, and strong abilities/verbal skills—may manage the shorter assignments and the less complex concepts of elementary school, many will have more academic difficulties in the upper grades in terms of quantity (longer assignments, more homework) and quality of work (increasingly abstract language and manipulating more complex ideas in their minds), as well as dealing with greater expectations to become more independent in their studies. Adolescents with ADHD frequently procrastinate, heeding Mark Twain's advice to "never put off until tomorrow what you can do the day after tomorrow." They may also do poorly on tests, be careless when doing their schoolwork, and have trouble tracking and turning in their assignments on time. Because they have more teachers in middle school and high school, there is a greater need for organizational skills. Proper medication treatment can go a long way in supporting your child's academic efforts. A treatment plan with specially targeted academic support at home and in the classroom is essential. It is also important to understand, however, that certain higher-level academic tasks, especially those requiring doing 2 or more things at the same time, may develop more slowly in your teenager with ADHD. This is not to say that your child can never do as well academically as his peers—only that he will probably have to work harder with structured individualized systems, strategies, and supports. Because there is no routine one-size-fits-all formula for these aids, your child may also need to rely on professional advice in designing the best routines and your own support, patience, and commitment.

A STUDENT'S STORY

Feeling Overwhelmed

"Last Thursday I forgot to take my pill. As the day progressed, I became increasingly distracted. By eighth period I could, for the first time, hear the low electrical buzz in the chemistry lab. I noticed the dripping of one of the faucets and the curled corner of a piece of paper peeling off of its poster board backing. I saw the faint streaks of green that lingered on the chalkboard beneath the white chalk equations. As a classmate's wisps of breath lightly touched my hair, I could feel the strands' small movements. Occasionally, I could discern fragments of conversation coming from the hall outside. As my head whirred with this overload of sensations the air seemed to congeal; grow slow. I felt heavy and lethargic; my senses seemed to have thickened and blurred. When class ended, I realized I had neglected to write down any of the directions for the next day's experiment.

I would often sit down and start my homework with the best of intentions. Two hours later I would look up and discover, to my surprise, that I had spent the whole time reading a 'few' chapters of a novel or staring out the window. I couldn't understand how I had lost that time!"

Sharon, Topeka, KS

As students mature, they are expected to be able to carry out more complex learning tasks—tasks that may prove especially challenging to your child with ADHD. These include

- **More consistent and sustained attention** to classroom lectures and deskwork
- **More efficient processing of information** encountered through reading or classroom lectures
- **Mature visual-spatial skills** that help interpret and reason
- **Complex thinking** that allows for advanced problem-solving and the ability to handle abstract concepts
- **Higher-level language abilities** required for a greater emphasis on abstract language and fluency in written language, as well as for studying a second language in school
- **Fine motor skills** needed for efficient note-taking, keyboard use, and speed writing
- **Better self-organization** needed to complete schoolwork each day and turn it in on time

- **Improved sequencing skills** to schedule enough time for schoolwork every day, plan the steps necessary to complete long-term assignments, prioritize work assignments, and keep up with school demands

This is a heavy menu of new demands for any student—especially those with ADHD and related problems. Delayed development of any of these skills can lead to poorer academic functioning. As your child moves toward adolescence, pay special attention to how well he is managing these types of challenges and plan to focus on them and put support systems into place as he continues to develop.

Reviewing Your Teenager's Education Program

Overseeing your child's academic career during adolescence is easier in some ways and more difficult in others. As your child matures, he is better able to communicate his school-related problems to you—though, as a teenager, he may be reluctant to do so. The fact that he attends multiple classes with a number of different teachers allows you to compare his performance among classes and therefore more accurately identify problems and needs. Teachers who now see him for just one period a day are less likely, however, to know your child well, and to be able to provide insight into his situation. Finally, while the chances are greater that by now you have been able to create structures and strategies that have worked for him over time, some problems may have been compounded by earlier failures, a decrease in self-esteem, the development of behavioral or emotional disorders, or an academic or social "reputation" that may be difficult to overcome.

As always, it is better to initially focus on your child's strengths, and only then to begin to tackle the weaknesses. If your teenager is having significant school problems and you have not already worked with school personnel to create an education program that meets his needs or considered seeking additional help for him under the Individuals with Disabilities Education Act (IDEA) or Section 504, refer to Chapter 7 for information on how to implement these sometimes vital forms of support. Particularly if your child is changing to a new school or you have not previously established contact with his principal or special education coordinator, meet with one of them now to discuss your teenager's diagnosis and any classroom accommodations that might be available if needed. If you feel that you need more support in this, ask your child's pediatrician to contact his school directly, and review Chapter 7 for ideas on other options.

Request a meeting with your child's educational team to help you prepare for the coming academic year. At this meeting (or, if no meeting is scheduled, during early conversations with as many of his teachers as possible once the school year has begun), find out when regular parent-teacher conferences are scheduled, arrange for additional regular meetings or phone conversations if you and the teacher agree that these would be helpful, and decide how to communicate about any issues that arise. Discuss how any special educational services or accommodations will be implemented. Arrange for the completion of a weekly report card if you have decided to use one. It is also a good idea to understand each teacher's philosophy concerning ADHD, and to tactfully correct any broad misconceptions. Emphasize from the start that you are there to support the teachers' efforts to help your teenager—not to second-guess the teachers or "tell them what to do."

After 2 or 3 months have passed, you, your child, and his teachers will have accumulated enough information about his performance to review a list of academic goals and, if necessary, revise his education program. Pay attention to the special skills he needs to develop to handle his increased workload, including

- Completing homework and turning it in on time
- Breaking down long-term assignments into manageable chunks and prioritizing daily assignments
- Comprehending and recalling what he reads
- Listening in class and taking adequate notes
- Memorizing facts
- Managing his time
- Organizing his study area, backpack, and class folders
- Writing legibly and quickly, and typing efficiently on a computer keyboard

Behavioral issues in the classroom should also be addressed at this time because they can strongly affect your teenager's ability to learn and the classroom environment in general. Teenagers with inattentive-type ADHD may especially need help in participating in class discussions or seeking extra help when they need it. Those with hyperactive-impulsive type

ADHD or a behavioral disorder are more likely to have problems with disrupting the class, arguing with teachers, getting into fights with classmates, or skipping class. Once you have identified the major functioning difficulties experienced by your child, and have prioritized them in order of importance, try to pinpoint exact targets for improvement. Does he have trouble memorizing facts because he tries to memorize too many in a single session? Does his disruptive behavior occur when quiet deskwork has gone on for longer than his patience allows, when school pressures (such as test taking) make him anxious, or when he has forgotten to take his medication?

Comparing your child's functioning from one classroom to another may add insight into precisely where a problem lies. If he is making As in math and Ds in history, for example, is it because his math teacher has a knack for keeping his attention or limiting his disruptive behavior? (If so, perhaps the math teacher would be willing to share his thoughts with others who teach your child.) Is it because special accommodations, such as untimed tests or shorter homework assignments, are provided in math class but not in history? Might he have an undiagnosed reading-related learning disability that is affecting his performance in history? Or is he simply passionate about math and less confident about history? (If so, his passion should be encouraged and his insecurity in other classes specifically addressed.) Does his schoolwork worsen in the late afternoon, and does this have anything to do with his medication beginning to wear off? Remember that adolescents with more intense needs may continue to qualify for Individualized Education Programs under IDEA and Section 504 of the Rehabilitation Act as discussed in Chapter 7.

Creating an Academic Contract

As adolescence progresses, it becomes increasingly important to assign your child more responsibility for implementing his own education program if he is to remain sufficiently motivated to follow it. One way to encourage your teenager's active participation is to create a "contract" to be signed by you, your child, and his teachers. Define the areas you have agreed to address, state how they will be addressed and who will be responsible for which actions, and specify the consequences (use of the family car, a later curfew on weekends) that your child will receive for successfully fulfilling the contract.

CREATING AN ACADEMIC CONTRACT

Contracts can be created for specific academic goals. If your teenager has difficulty studying for tests, for example, his contract might read

- Your teacher will go over material that will be on an upcoming test, clearly state the date of the test at least a week in advance, and write the date on the chalkboard.
- You will
  1. Study for the test for 30 minutes each weekday for 1 week using the study techniques you have been taught.
  2. Spend 10 minutes each day with your academic coach or tutor reviewing the material you have studied that day.
  3. Communicate with your teacher before the test if you feel the need to take the test untimed.
  4. After the test, review these strategies with me or your coach to judge which ones worked and which ones did not.
  5. Revise the study plan for the next test on the basis of the review.
- If the 5 steps are completed, you will be able to stay out an extra hour on weekend nights for the following month (a prenegotiated privilege).

Keep in mind that this contract only specifies the processes that he will follow, not the grades that he receives.

A signed contract communicates to your teenager his "adult" role in managing his own academic progress and spells out precisely how he can take control of his success. Teenagers who do not see the connection between their own actions and their academic successes or failures are more likely to experience school failure. By literally outlining the steps your child can take to change his own situation, and mapping out how you and his teachers will support him in getting where he wants to go, you can foster his chances of succeeding and his need for independence at the same time.

Specific Schoolwork Strategies

One of the best ways to teach your teenager the skills he will need to succeed in school is to break complex processes down into a series of simpler steps. In many cases, teenagers with ADHD fail to succeed at school because they simply do not know how to study effectively for tests, keep their school notebooks organized, or plan for more complex assignments—

processes that we call *executive functions.* These techniques are not always easy to develop naturally. You can certainly share the strategies that *you* use with your teenager—*but remember* that what works for you will not necessarily work for him. You can also ask your child's teacher or school counselor to refer you to a tutor who can problem-solve with your teenager to find his own most effective ways to memorize material, more fully comprehend what he reads, study for tests, organize his backpack, manage his homework assignments, or accomplish whatever other school related tasks you have identified. The teacher or counselor may also be able to contribute valuable ideas. Some teenagers with ADHD also find it quite helpful to find peer tutoring programs and study-skills classes if they are available in their schools. Study and time management tips are also available on most ADHD-related Web sites, including www.add.org and www.chadd.org. In most cases, such instruction requires only a few brief sessions. You can then follow up on this instruction at home with your child.

GOOD HABITS FOR ACADEMIC SUCCESS

Helping your teenager to discover the tools and motivation to organize his life can make an immense difference in his academic progress and, in turn, his self-esteem. Here are some tips that he may find useful. But remember, study habits need to be individualized, and what works well for one person may not for another.

- **Keep the organization simple.** Consider keeping just one folder for all work that is completed, another folder for all work that still needs to be done, and a third folder for graded work and notes from the teacher to the parents. When your student gets home, he can pull out one folder containing all the assignments he needs to complete. At the end of the evening, all of these assignments will have been placed in the completed work folder. At the end of the next school day the completed work folder should be empty, because all the work has been turned in. Complicated systems like color coding each folder for each subject may seem like a better idea, but can become overwhelming for many students with ADHD. Consider that more complicated organizing systems may be better but work best for students who are already well organized.

- **Use a daily planner or handheld computer** to record school assignments, doctor's appointments, and other meetings, and to schedule work on long-term projects. Again, keep it simple. Elaborate systems may be more detailed but more frustrating to use.

GOOD HABITS FOR ACADEMIC SUCCESS (CONTINUED)

- **Use a backpack as the location for all schoolwork and supplies.** Supplies can be kept in the side pockets, his assignment planner in a separate outside pocket, and his notebook in the main body of the pack. All schoolwork goes into the backpack.

- **Organize an assigned locker** as a place to keep schoolbooks not needed that day—not as a trash can or repository for supplies and papers.

- **Make lists** of tasks to be accomplished, ideas to be included in a written essay, people to call about a project, etc. The more short-term information a teenager has on paper, the less he has to hold in his head. Keep the lists in a designated place (a computer, a backpack, a "note box" at home, etc). Lists scattered throughout the house can be harder to find than remembering the information they contain.

- **Use an outline or flowchart format to take notes.** An outline or flowchart can help a teenager understand the structure underlying the information he hears and can save him from having to write down every word.

- **Preview.** If there are questions in the back of a chapter in a textbook, reading these questions first can help students know ahead of time what major points the author thinks he should take away from the chapter.

- **Break up large tasks into a series of small steps.** Study for tests in a series of relatively brief periods over a number of days instead of cramming the night before. Good study habits can include surveying the topics to be tested; creating questions about the material, then rereading the material to answer his questions; formulating answers in his head or discussing them with you, a tutor, or a "study buddy"; and practicing writing down answers to questions that seem likely to be on the test. He could plan a writing assignment by doing the research one day, thinking about it the next, writing a first draft on the third day, and revising it on the fourth.

- **Set aside a routine time and place for doing homework.** Most teenagers with ADHD can benefit from a routine, non-distracting environment for completing work. This may mean no television or Internet access unless it is required for an assignment.

GOOD HABITS FOR ACADEMIC SUCCESS (CONTINUED)

- **Take advantage of his learning style.** A teenager should pay attention to how he learns best. Is it easier for him to memorize by using abbreviations or acronyms (making a word from the first letter of each memorized term), looking at lists or charts, reviewing facts verbally with a partner, or testing and retesting himself on paper? Does he work better in short bursts or for longer periods? Alone or with others present? In his room or at the dining table?

- **Create "bypass" strategies.** Teenagers with uneven learning styles can benefit from developing bypass strategies—strategies designed to help work around a particular problem. For example, if a student gets overwhelmed by a long-term assignment because of extreme difficulty with handwriting, a bypass strategy would be to get permission to use a computer. If a student has extreme difficulty "multitasking" (writing while thinking) and, because of this, loses track of his thoughts, it may be helpful to first dictate several ideas into a computer or tape recorder and then write them down, separating the 2 tasks and making each one more doable.

Consider that all of the suggestions above are not one size fits all. Some may be successful and others not. Some of them can be easily used as stated, others may have to be adapted to your adolescent's learning style to be helpful.

Social and Emotional Challenges in Adolescence

Most teenagers have concerns about being accepted by their peers, but many teens with ADHD have come to expect some social rejection due to their difficulties with controlling their behavior and understanding others' social signals. Social issues encountered in childhood can become worse in adolescence, with the intensity of any rejection or bullying increasing during the teenage years. This rejection can negatively affect both academic performance and emotional health—and can be, in fact, much more troubling to him than making poor grades in school. He also may appear emotionally immature compared with classmates, and sometimes he'll be more comfortable interacting with younger peers or when spending time with adults who may show greater acceptance of his immature actions.

As with academic challenges, however, difficulties with social interaction can often be helped by having adolescents learn specific skills. In chapters 5 and 6, you learned a number of ways to teach younger children how to interact positively with others, including role modeling, role-playing, analyzing interaction, and practicing new techniques. Now, in adolescence, your child is likely to experience new motivation to improve his social life, and advice about social issues is now more often sought from peers than from parents.

Friendships

Teenagers with ADHD can certainly have the close friendships that are important for their happiness and self-esteem. A teenager's targeted efforts to increase the accuracy of his social perceptions and monitor his social interactions may make this easier for him. As he develops friendships, support this by allowing his friends to hang out in your home and help to provide the kind of supportive environment that facilitates all friendships. Observe how the friends relate to one another, and provide tactful feedback later if you feel that it will be received in a positive and constructive manner. Teenagers with ADHD need to be increasingly aware that friendships take organizational skills too—returning phone calls, arriving at meeting places on time, and following through on plans.

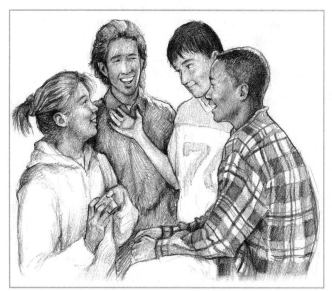

Teenagers with ADHD certainly can have the close friendships that are important for their happiness and self-esteem.

Conflict Resolution

It is important for your teenager to learn how to resolve conflict without resorting to physical fights, and how to avoid becoming the target of others' aggression. Again, resolving conflict can be a difficult teenage task if his impulsiveness causes him to strike out when he gets upset. An important step in avoiding this problem is to identify his own anger cues and to brainstorm in advance about the kinds of positive solutions he can apply to future conflicts. If this is an issue with your teenager, through discussions with you and peers; post-conflict analysis; and sessions with a counselor, therapist, or social-skills instructor, he can learn to "talk himself down" when he finds himself in a frustrating clash of wills ("I'm going to take three deep breaths and think about my best choice in this situation before lashing out."). He can also practice conflict-prevention techniques, such as providing an alternative ("How about if we go bowling first and then see a movie?"), adding provisions ("OK, you can drive, but then I get to decide on the restaurant."), or changing the subject ("I'm starving. You want to get some pizza?"). Once your child has learned a few of these specific techniques, he may be surprised at how effective they are in helping him avoid the crises that used to disrupt his social life. If you are seeking counseling in this area, the most proven approach is through cognitive-behavioral therapy—this is a type of talk therapy that views behavioral issues as related to the interaction of thoughts, behaviors, and emotions. In cognitive-behavioral therapy, the therapist and adolescent will work on identifying and directly changing behaviors that are problematic.

Working on Social Skills

As with other learning processes, your teenager can hone his social skills and interaction by

- Developing a list of specific target behaviors to work on
- Outlining a step-by-step plan to address each one
- Receiving consistent, tactful feedback from you, his peers, and his teachers
- Learning such techniques as identifying cues that set off his anger, analysis of others' social interaction, social role-playing, etc
- Getting training in anger management or social skills, or treatment in individual or group therapy, when appropriate
- Receiving treatment for any coexisting conditions that may affect his social interaction (See Chapter 9.)
- Getting positive feedback for improvement in targeted social skills
- Staying involved in rewarding prosocial activities

That said, it is also true that many people with ADHD continue to have trouble with certain social interactions throughout adolescence and into adulthood. Whether or not this is the case with your teenager, make it clear that you support him no matter what. Nothing will be more difficult for him than overcoming social rejection. It will mean a lot to your teenager to know that you will always be in his corner. Keep in mind that even teenagers who are socially unhappy in high school go on to find rewarding friendships in college or work situations.

Your Teenager's Emotional Development

It is easy to see how academic, social, and family strains can create a heavy emotional burden for adolescents with ADHD. Low self-esteem caused by academic failure and social rejection can lead to depression, defensiveness, pessimism about the future, hostility, and physical aggression. Combined with ADHD-related impulsiveness, it can pave the way for unsafe sexual activity; alcohol, tobacco, or drug abuse; and other high-risk behavior. Take a moment to consider your teenager's emotional state. Does he spend nearly all of his time alone in his room? Does he seem sad nearly all the time, or irritable? Is his anger starting to get out of hand? Has he been suspended from school more than once this year, or are you receiving reports of inappropriate behavior? If so, discuss these issues with your adolescent and bring them up at follow-up sessions with his pediatrician. Anxiety and depressive disorders (see Chapter 9) are prominent coexisting conditions in teenagers with ADHD, and should be thought of any time an adolescent's social, academic, or behavioral functioning starts to deteriorate without an obvious explanation. In teenage years depression and anxiety increase significantly in individuals with ADHD. Whereas in childhood the number of boys and girls who experience depression are about equal, in adolescence the number of girls outnumber boys by 2 to 1. The sooner an adolescent's depression, anxiety, anger, substance use, etc, is recognized, the greater the chances that the situation can be resolved before worse problems develop.

Risk Taking

Adolescence is a time when all teenagers are prone to testing limits and engaging in risk taking. Adolescents with ADHD and an impulsive style are especially prone to taking risks. Surveys have shown that teenagers with ADHD can have an earlier age of first intercourse, more partners, less use of birth control, and more sexually transmitted infections and teenage pregnancy than their peers. Education about these issues in the preteen years and continuing guidance now can really pay off.

Driving can be a particular area of concern as well. Teenage drivers with ADHD have been reported to be 8 times more likely to lose their license, 4 times more likely to be involved in a collision, 3 times more likely to sustain a serious injury, and 2 to 4 times more likely to receive a moving violation. As a parent, you may want to consider this area carefully, make sure that your adolescent is at a maturity level appropriate for driving, and set appropriate limits if necessary. Some parents restrict the time of day when their adolescent with ADHD can drive and make driving contingent on responsible driving behavior. It is a known fact that teenage driving accidents go up progressively with the number of people in the car. Parents may put limits on how many teenagers can travel in the car when your teenager is behind the wheel, particularly in the first year or two of driving. Discuss safe driving at home. Where medication is found helpful in cutting down on impulsivity, it makes sense to have a rule that teenagers who respond well to medication make sure that their medication schedule includes driving times. Finally, as with any teenager it makes ultimate sense to have a "parent taxi" understanding. Even if use of alcohol or drugs is never condoned by parents, develop an understanding that it is always safe for your teenager to call you and ask you to pick them up if they are even minimally impaired from these substances.

Effective Parenting of Teenagers With ADHD

In chapters 5 and 6, you learned of a number of parenting techniques aimed at helping you interact positively with your younger child. These behavior management techniques can still provide a basis for healthy family relationships, but as your teenager grows increasingly independent you will need to deal with more complex family issues that require some new approaches. A number of these issues are discussed in this section, along with some effective techniques you can use to address them. As when your child was younger, however, you are likely to benefit enormously from sound parenting education information specially designed for families of teenagers with ADHD, or from the counseling of a therapist trained in these techniques.

Helping Your Teenager Become More Independent

As you have learned, achieving independence is every adolescent's primary developmental goal. Your teenager will experience this urge as strongly as his peers without ADHD, but his impulsivity, inattention, and aspects of delayed maturation mean that he may need to move more slowly toward full self-supervision. Specifically, you may need to

- Remove limits and loss of privileges at as rapid a pace as possible, as your adolescent shows that he can take responsibility. Long-standing loss of privileges harbors resentment and has little teaching value.
- Work harder at consciously modeling responsible behavior.
- Break down tasks and responsibilities into smaller steps and reward him systematically for accomplishing them.
- Develop a plan for systematically transferring responsibilities over to your teenager as he works on his own independence.

In short, sensitive monitoring and limit setting will be critical as your teenager works his way toward mature self-management and autonomy.

Of course, any adolescent would resent a 10:00 pm curfew, for example, if his friends are allowed to stay out until midnight. You should address your concerns directly—talk with him about the reasons if you worry about his staying out later. You may be concerned that parties tend to get wilder after about 10:00 pm, a time where you have observed that his impulsivity usually increases, or that driving is potentially riskier late at night because his medication will have worn off by then. If he counters that he is ready to take responsibility for staying out later, and you believe that this may be true and have made the necessary adjustments to ensure success (in this case possibly changing his dosage routine to enhance attention while driving), extend the curfew for 1 hour. If he arrives home on time with no evidence of high-risk activity, praise him and reward him with a continued 11:00 pm curfew. Moving in these smaller steps allows you to continue to systematically build on these successes while giving him the chance to extend the boundaries of his independence. Such triumphs in mutual trust and respect are vital for a teenager's self-esteem and positive attitude.

Providing Structure and Support

During your child's earlier years, you were encouraged to actively monitor his behavior in the classroom and at home, providing frequent rewards and, when necessary, punishments. Now that your teenager is growing more independent, you may feel it is time to stop this type of monitoring. However, many teenagers with ADHD continue to need more parental monitoring and structure than their peers without ADHD. While it is best for parents of many other 15-year-olds to back off and let their child manage his own homework production, for instance, adolescents with ADHD may need continued monitoring to see that he is completing his work and turning it in on time. While other parents may grow more lax about knowing where their older teenagers are every minute, you may have reason to continue monitoring where your teenager is, with whom, what he is doing, and when he will be home, particularly when you sense that he might find himself in a high-risk situation that may be difficult for him to manage. This must be done, however, in a manner respectful of your teenager and his developmental needs.

Establishing and Enforcing Rules

Teenagers with ADHD may have an argumentative style, and your teenager's resistance to your continued monitoring is likely to lead to a great deal of boundary testing, negotiating, and possibly outright rebellion. When warranted, you may feel better—and will be able to save some energy—if you identify 4 or 5 *nonnegotiable* rules based on the issues you consider essential for your family. You may decide, for example, that use of illegal drugs of any kind—including marijuana, alcohol, and cigarettes—will not be tolerated in your house, or that driving can only be done at times when stimulant medication still has an active effect. These strict, nonnegotiable rules should be reserved for critical issues of safety or family functioning.

When you have arrived at the 4 or 5 basic rules, write them down and discuss them with your teenager. Explain that the trust built through compliance with these rules can open the door to negotiating the other freedoms he craves. His efforts to respect these few bottom-line demands will improve communication and pave the way toward that greater trust. Finally (and this part can be negotiated), discuss with him the rewards for compliance (extended privileges in other areas) and the consequences (increased restrictions) for breaking these rules, and then enforce these consequences consistently.

Negotiating With Your Adolescent

Once your teenager has agreed to follow these few essential rules, you are likely to feel more at ease when negotiating other issues with him. As the parent of an adolescent with ADHD, you will need to become adept at using negotiation to shape behavior and to resolve conflicts as they occur, while at the same time respecting his need for independence. Negotiation is based on the assumption that, as an adolescent matures, he will take a more active role in creating the rules by which he lives. While your goal should be to gradually lead him toward a thoughtful independence in managing his behavior, it is important to establish the fact that as the parent, right now you assume the final responsibility for rules and consequences around selective critical issues.

A good way to negotiate rules or solutions to family conflicts is to use a technique called problem-solving training. This technique consists of the following steps:

- Define the problem and its effect.
- Come up with a variety of possible solutions to the problem.
- Choose the best solution.
- Plan how to implement the solution.
- Renegotiate a new solution if necessary.

Your teenager may resent the fact that he is not allowed to watch television on school nights, for example. To resolve this conflict, you could hold a family meeting to discuss the issue. First, you would *define the problem* and allow him to explain why it upsets him. ("Steven, you want to watch three to four hours of TV on weeknights like you say all your friends are doing," and then you might add, "but I see that when you do that you usually only get about half of your homework finished." Steven might respond, "Everybody talks about what they watched the night before, and I never have anything to say. It makes me feel left out and like a loser.")

Next you, your partner, and your teenager would *contribute ideas to resolve this problem.*

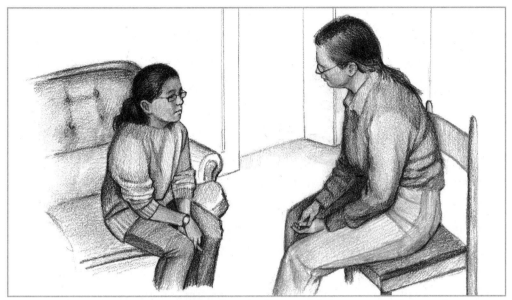

As a parent of an adolescent with ADHD you will need to become skilled at using negotiation to shape your child's behavior and resolve conflicts as they occur.

Usually 6 to 8 ideas are sufficient. No one should express judgment or respond to any of the suggestions in any way, positively or negatively. Each family member should contribute whatever solution comes to mind, even if it seems somewhat unusual or impractical—taking turns, if necessary, to allow each person to contribute his or her share. Your adolescent or you should write down each potential solution until all suggestions have been recorded.

Next, each family member should take a turn *evaluating* each solution in order. He should consider whether a particular solution would work for him, whether it would work for others in the family, and then assign it a plus or a minus. As the family works down the list of solutions in this way, each solution will accumulate a series of plus and/or minus ratings that can be used to choose the best idea.

To choose a solution, you and your family can select any idea that has received all "pluses" and discuss its benefits and weaknesses. If more than one solution has received all pluses, you might be able to pick the one that seems most reasonable to your adolescent. If none has received unanimous approval, choose the one that was best liked and discuss how you might make it acceptable or brainstorm again to find a solution acceptable to everyone. (For a solution to work well, it needs to create a "win-win" situation.) In this way, you will end up with a solution that you can all live with—even if none of you consider it perfect.

Once you have chosen the best solution, you will need to agree on *how it will be implemented.* Who will be responsible for seeing that rules are followed? Who will remind your teenager to comply with the rules when necessary? What are the consequences for breaking the rules and the rewards for complying? If you have agreed, for example, that Steven can watch television for 1 hour each school night as long as he has completed his homework, you must jointly decide how late at night he can watch television, who will be responsible for reminding him that his homework needs to be finished first, who will check to make sure it is done, what privileges he will lose if he breaks these rules, and what rewards he will enjoy if he follows them. The more airtight you can make this part of the agreement, the less time and energy you will spend arguing about the rules later. The entire agreement should be written down and, if appropriate, signed by everyone present.

When first attempting to solve problems in this way, it is best to start with issues that are important but not emotionally intense for your teenager or for you. Once you have practiced these new techniques with one or more easier topics, you can move toward resolving more volatile conflicts. Eventually you may become so adept at this rational form of problem-solving that you and your teenager will be able to resolve arguments on the spot, in most cases, using informal versions of this technique.

Providing Appropriate Consequences

Throughout this book, we have emphasized the importance of providing positive reinforcement whenever possible, ignoring negative behaviors that are not dangerous or destructive, and punishing only the few intolerable behaviors on which you and your child are currently focusing. This practice should continue throughout adolescence—with the reminder that the more positive feedback you can offer your child during these difficult years, the more competent he is likely to feel. It is also a fact that you will need to save consequences or other negative feedback for the times when you really need them. Constant criticism or punishment will desensitize your child to your reactions, so that he may not respond if you ever get truly angry or concerned.

You will need to "stick to your guns" in enforcing the rules and procedures on which you have all already agreed. Provide rewards and consequences consistently, and as soon as possible after the behavior has occurred. Measures such as time-outs are no longer age-appropriate for adolescents. More appropriate consequences include pre–agreed-on losses of privileges, such as temporarily losing car key rights for coming home late. Try to let these negotiated consequences take the place of argument, recrimination, yelling, or nitpicking. Keeping the conflicts and emotions out of it, and simply providing the appropriate response, is one way to keep family life relatively pleasant and upbeat.

Fostering a Positive Attitude and Giving Each Other Breaks

Your support and sensitive parenting can make all the difference to an adolescent who may meet with rejection, frustration, or even failure at school. Research suggests, in fact, that the presence of one fully supportive adult in the life of a child with ADHD is one of the key factors in determining that child's future success. Be sure to invest plenty of quality time in your teenager—and make it fun and rewarding for both of you. Sometimes, when things get too tough at home, it is a good idea to take a break from one another. A weekend that you spend away can restore your awareness that your problems at home can be solved, and can give all of you the space you need to maintain a healthy relationship. Parents need support too!

Adolescence is an exciting period. It is a time of exploration and emerging independence, the transition from childhood to adulthood. This can be both a highly rewarding and tumultuous journey. As any teenager explores newly accessible choices, he or she will inevitably make some good and bad decisions. This is a normal and important part of becoming a responsible adult. As your family negotiates this developmental stage, it pays to keep in mind that your adolescent is a teenager first, and a teenager with ADHD somewhere down the line. Allowing this exploration is a critical element for arriving at the other end as a capable, responsible adult.

Q & A

Q: When our son was first diagnosed with ADHD at age 9, my husband and I worked hard to put a consistent system of rewards and consequences in place to help him manage his behavior. Now that he's 13, however, he's gotten very good at circumventing one parent's rules by getting the other to agree to concessions, and even just ignoring the limits we've set. For the first time this year, he was suspended from school for behavior issues, and we're afraid things might be getting worse. Are we doing something wrong?

A: First, it is important to remember that nearly all adolescents test behavioral limits and experiment with how best to circumvent parental rules. That said, it is especially important during these years that you remain as consistent as possible when discussing, setting, and enforcing a behavioral "bottom line." Talk seriously with your teenager about the reasons why he needs to follow certain rules. It becomes more and more important at this age to make sure that he agrees that the consequences and rewards are fair to him—but negotiate these beforehand and not in the heat of battle. Make sure you and your partner are presenting him with a united front—allowing him to play one of you against another is one of the easiest traps that parents fall into. If you feel that he believes there may be no consequences to his behavior, consider creating a written contract for all of you to sign, stipulating the rules to be followed and related rewards and punishments. Keep in mind that teenagers with ADHD can be impulsive, and many find that it is difficult to keep their behavior within tolerable limits. However, where impulsive behaviors in grade school may have included pushing in line and blurting out answers before the teacher finished asking the question, impulsivity in teenagers can include high-risk behaviors leading to drug use, teenage pregnancy, serious conduct problems, and school dropout. This makes it particularly important to develop a parenting style that includes your adolescent in the decision-making; leads to good self-esteem; and includes setting firm, but also sensitive and fair, limits when appropriate.

Q: Our 14-year-old daughter, who has inattentive-type ADHD, has changed completely over the past 6 months. Her grades, which used to be Bs and Cs, were nearly all Ds and Fs this past semester, and she spends almost all her free time locked in her room. We've met with her and her teachers about the grades and she's promised to work to get them up, but I haven't seen her changing her behavior much at all since then. Is this a normal part of being a teenager, or should we be concerned?

A: An abrupt change in behavior and declining grades are 2 warning signs that any teenager—and especially an adolescent with ADHD—needs help. The behaviors you describe could be signs of depression, anxiety, substance abuse, or a serious decline in self-esteem caused by social or other problems. Any sudden changes in behavior that lead to a decline in functioning should be considered "red flags" and evaluated. Because adolescents are so concerned with independence, your daughter may not be able to ask you for help directly, but may be actually expecting you to interpret behaviors, such as locking herself in her room, as a cry for help. Far from being considered negative, by pursuing these concerns and setting up an evaluation you are also conveying a powerful message of support to her.

Chapter 12

A Look at Your Child's Future

Most children and teenagers with attention-deficit/hyperactivity disorder (ADHD) find the elementary school and high school years difficult in one way or another. New challenges emerge as your child reaches the end of adolescence and looks forward to a more independent life of his own. Whether he goes straight from high school into a job or attends college, he will need to continue to monitor any ongoing functioning problems related to ADHD, advocate effectively for his needs, and structure his life in ways that will help him succeed. Why? Because between one-half to two-thirds of children with ADHD will continue to have some significant symptoms as adults. To help your teen as he transitions to more independent living you will need to assume new roles and assist in his acquisition of a set of skills to ensure success. Since your child will likely grow up with increasingly more effective treatment methods than are presently available, he is also likely to have an even better outcome than the current research suggests. In this chapter, you will find helpful information on

- How to help your child research and apply to colleges and universities that can satisfy his interests and needs
- How he can best transition to life as a young adult in college or in a job
- Health and safety issues of special importance to adults with ADHD
- Relationship challenges and family responsibilities that your grown child will need to learn to manage
- Current and future research that may help your child live more successfully with ADHD in the years ahead

After High School: College and Work

Your teenager can best prepare himself for this giant step toward independence by thinking about what sort of adult life he hopes to have. Whether he chooses a pathway of a work or a college experience, he will need to continue to develop life-management skills (executive functions) that include the abilities to organize, plan, prioritize, curb acting on impulses, and stick to plans, but also be able to know when they need to be altered. Developing these skills is often difficult for individuals who have ADHD, but are very much required for independent living. Teens who have worked on these skills during high school—money management, time management, planning, daily life maintenance skills—will need to continue to develop these skills in the workplace or in college.

Has your teenager with ADHD been frustrated by the work demands of his high school environment and longed for the time when he can run his own life and be his own boss? Does he have a special passion or talent that occupies much of his energy and attention? This may be the time to explore his interests more deeply through an internship, apprenticeship, or entry-level job. Are a higher education and professional job prospects important to him?

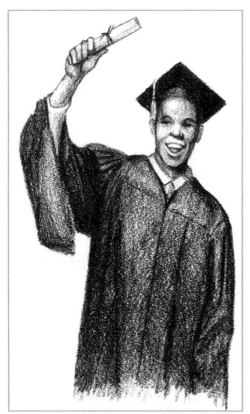

Talk frequently with your teenager about his special passion, talent, or interest. This can help him think about what sort of adult life he hopes to have.

Then he should consider attending college—and may want to take advantage of special programs designed to help students with ADHD. Of course, no high school student can be expected to come up with a definitive answer to all of these questions right away, but it is important to at least start to consider them before jumping into a first job or higher-education experience. Frequent job and career changes are one reason why some adults with ADHD lag behind their peers in career success. Thinking things out carefully and resisting the impulse to "act first and think later" may save time and effort in the long run.

High school is also the time to work on the skills needed to be successful at college and in life. Is your teen able to take care of his daily living needs? Can he get himself up in the morning and get himself to bed at night at a reasonable hour? Is he able to manage his own laundry and other personal needs? Can he take responsibility for his medication and treatment programs by making his own appointments at the doctor and call for his prescriptions? How are his organization and time-management skills? Can he create a schedule for all assignments and plan his after-school schedule? It's also time to take a look at your role in your teen's development. If your teen is still overly dependent on you for many of these critical life skills, it may be time to set up a program that allows your teen to grow and take on more responsibilities while he is still at home.

Once your teenager has begun working on the various skills needed for a successful launch into adulthood, the next step is thinking about whether he wants to attend college immediately after high school or if another path would be better suited for him. His high school counselor can be a valuable resource in this process. A good counselor can provide him with an objective picture of his school and learning profile and discuss with him how his interests best match different jobs and occupations, where their typical stresses and satisfactions lie, and how he might find a satisfying path toward his career goal. If he has had an ongoing Individualized Education Program (IEP), the counselor can also help see that the types of post–secondary school transition steps mandated by the Individuals with Disabilities Education Act (IDEA) (see box on page 290) are being carried out effectively for him. Your teenager should also discuss his plans for the future with his pediatrician, psychologist, psychiatrist, or other medical advisor, particularly in terms of how his ADHD symptoms may affect his experiences in various jobs and professions, and how he can continue to effectively monitor and self-manage his symptoms.

Thinking About College

Choosing an appropriate school is difficult for most college-bound students, but it can become an even more complicated process, and more crucial, for a teenager with ADHD. Not only must he find a college that suits his academic, social, and geographical preferences, but he also must decide whether the education format and any special services provided by the institution will be sufficient to support his needs. Your adolescent, even more than many of his peers, may need to ask himself "Is this the right fit for me?" in addition to the universal cry of "Will I be accepted?"

Teens often are unaware of how different college is from high school in academic as well as other areas. No one will be there to make sure he attends classes, completes his assignments, or even accesses services. In addition, many of the services students are accustomed to receiving in high school may not be available at college. Self-knowledge and a good transition plan are important to ensure success at the college level.

TRANSITION PLANS: PREPARING FOR THE FUTURE

The IDEA stipulates that, from about age 14 years, when a youth with ADHD enters high school, his IEP team should start to discuss and consider his goals for post-school adult life. By age 16 years or even earlier, if appropriate, the IEP must include a statement of the transition services your child will need—that is, services that will facilitate his progress toward his career, academic, or other aspirations. Such services may include preparation for Scholastic Aptitude Tests (SATs) or other proficiency tests necessary when applying for college admission, as well as training in self-advocacy and self-sufficiency skills.

During your child's junior and senior years of high school, he should be reassessed for specific functioning problems related to his ADHD, learning disabilities, and any other coexisting conditions—particularly if he plans to attend college. He will need to provide detailed documentation of these disabilities to qualify for untimed or other special college-entry testing accommodations and for special support services at college. His IEP alone, or a general diagnosis of ADHD, will not be sufficient to obtain these services.

Once your child graduates from high school, he will no longer receive services provided by the school system. However, if he has been receiving services, such as counseling and vocational evaluation and assessment, as part of his transition plan, he can continue to receive them. An Individual Written Rehabilitation Plan (IWRP) will be created for him, allowing him to take advantage of such services.

Not every student with ADHD will need a formal transition plan, an IEP, or an IWRP. However, a well thought out plan that touches on the same themes will still be important. For more information on this and other aspects of preparing for life after graduation, consult your child's school guidance counselor, as well as www.add.org, www.chadd.org, www.pacer.org, and other responsible Web sites serving students and adults with ADHD.

What to Look for in Post-secondary Education

Location, size, and academic offerings are 3 important elements for all prospective students to consider when choosing among the many colleges available to them—and these are vital areas of concern for your teenager as well. He will need to think about whether he prefers to attend school near home, allowing him to take advantage of familiar resources, or farther away where he can "start his own life"—understanding, however, that he will continue to need the support that allowed him to be successful enough to get into college in the first place and that he may have to identify and make contact with a new set of medical and support services at his new school. He must consider which is better for him: a small college, where personal attention may be easier to obtain, or a large university with possibly better funding and more options for support services. He must also decide whether the institution's academic demands and supports will match his learning style and needs.

Because the transition to a self-structured life outside the home can be especially challenging for teenagers with ADHD, it is critical that your teen be well-prepared for life on his own. He will need to know and explain to others his various strengths and weaknesses as well as be willing to access services on his own. While the presence and effectiveness of a college's ADHD support program is a prime consideration, your teen must be mature enough to know if he needs to access the program. A few colleges specialize in educating students with learning disabilities. Others offer comprehensive support systems with trained, experienced staff and many specialized services for students with ADHD. Most offer limited specialized services and accommodations for students with ADHD, while some provide only a single learning center serving all students with disabilities and students who need temporary tutoring. The quality of support services offered by a college or university may outweigh considerations and preferences in other areas. Family discussions, for example, may conclude that a large or geographically distant university may work as a first choice if its support services are stronger than those of a college closer to home.

COLLEGE SUPPORT SERVICES AND ACCOMMODATIONS

Before he can choose an appropriate college, your teenager will need to consider—ideally with you and his guidance counselor, teachers, pediatrician, and/or psychologist—which services or accommodations he may need in his new life as an undergraduate. Services and accommodations for college students with ADHD may include

- **Special orientation programs** to introduce students to the institution's academic structure and available services
- **Specialized academic advisors or counselors** to help students identify the classes, professors, class load, and even the major best suited to their interests and needs
- **Priority scheduling** to allow students to sign up for the most appropriate classes at the most appropriate times of day
- **Reduced course loads,** which prevents students with ADHD from becoming overwhelmed (A reduced course load may mean that the student will have to make up credits during summer school or a fifth year.)
- **A private dormitory room** for students who may find the presence of a roommate too distracting or disruptive
- **Math laboratories, writing workshops, computer laboratories, and reading courses** to supplement and improve basic academic skills
- **Specialized tutoring** for students with ADHD—emphasizing organizational and planning skills and effective study techniques, as well as help with specific coursework and examination preparation
- **A "personal coach"** to check in with the student each day, reviewing his schedule for the day and the work she expects to accomplish
- **Classroom technology,** such as laptop computers, tape recorders, videos, and other recording aids, to facilitate students' ability to retain and review the information in classroom lectures
- **Academic aides,** including in-class note-takers and homework editors
- **Special testing arrangements,** such as untimed examinations or testing in a separate, quiet room
- **Advocates** to help communicate a student's diagnosis and needs to professors when appropriate and to help him obtain needed services
- **Support groups** or contact with other students with ADHD who can provide companionship, emotional support, and information
- **Career guidance and mentoring** for students with ADHD

Once your teenager has identified the services that are high priorities for him, he can look for colleges and universities that provide those services. Support services are not always described in college catalogs and brochures, so you and your teenager may need to do some extra research to find out exactly what is available at each institution. The first step for you or your teenager is to call or visit the special services office of each institution that interests him to determine which services may be available at that college or university. (The actual name of the services office tends to vary by institution. It may be listed as "student disability services," "learning support services," or something similar.) Early contact and familiarization with the student support office is important because this office is most often responsible for notifying professors about any classroom accommodations to which a student is entitled. Once enrolled at the college, students must register with the office and provide documentation of their disability to receive special services.

Some students, however, may choose to start college without ever disclosing their ADHD diagnosis, or they may decide to disclose it to the special services office only when they feel they would benefit from the types of services described previously. The choice of whether and when to disclose this information is highly individual, but deserves thought and discussion as your adolescents begin their college search. There is certainly no right or wrong approach, but students with obvious and ongoing support needs might more strongly consider exploring support services at the time that they begin thinking about college.

Following is a list of general questions that your teenager may want to present to the representative of each college's special services office. Of course, he will want to tailor the questions to apply to his particular anticipated needs. He may obtain more helpful information by also providing the representative with a list of the accommodations or services he hopes to obtain, along with documentation supporting his diagnosis of ADHD and his need for particular aids.

- What services or accommodations does the university or college routinely provide for students with ADHD—for example, specialized academic advising, early registration, a private dormitory room, untimed testing, or any of the other services listed previously? Is there an extra charge for any of these services? If the college does not provide them, are they conveniently available off campus?

- How long has the support services office existed? How many, if any, staff members are specially trained to work with students who have ADHD?
- How many students with ADHD does the office serve?
- Does the university provide other services for all students that may especially benefit students with ADHD—such as Web-based services that provide lecture notes or videos online, small seminars to review material covered in classroom lectures, and a willingness to work with new instructional techniques or technology?
- Are academic counselors or psychologists available on an ongoing basis to help students with ADHD adjust to college life and help with any problems that arise?
- Do counselors help connect students with faculty members who are knowledgeable and supportive regarding the needs of students with ADHD? Is there a program in place to educate faculty members about ADHD?
- Do support groups for students with ADHD exist on campus? Can the office provide your child with the names of other students with ADHD who are willing to be contacted?

Another consideration is that some youth with ADHD are slower to mature, so that starting at a local junior college with your child living at home may provide a more gradual opportunity for him to adjust to the college environment and be better able to adjust to the challenges of attending college away from home and the supports you have probably put in place to help facilitate his success in school up to now. Some students who have started college may find a need to return to the family nest—letting parents know that it's difficult for them to develop the life-management skills that independent living requires, particularly in the context of the freedom of college or living separately. This may provide them the opportunity to further build these skills as well as their self-esteem, and be in a better position to re-enter and be more successful in college academic and social life.

How to Apply

Once your adolescent has created a short list of colleges that best suit his interests and needs, he will begin the application process. Most colleges and universities require applicants to take Scholastic Aptitude Tests (SATs) or American College Testing (ACT) examinations. A student with ADHD can apply to take these tests under extended time conditions or with other special accommodations. To do this, he must present a written diagnosis of his condition, signed by a qualified, appropriate professional (dated or updated within the past 3 years) along with evidence of early impairment, current impairment, and specific problems. In addition, he will need a copy of his IEP at school and proof that he receives testing accommodations at school similar to those he is presently requesting. Because further documentation and possibly testing by a psychologist may be required, and specific dates are reserved for special testing, your teenager should contact the Web sites of the Educational Testing Service, the organization that administers the SAT examinations, at www.ets.org, or the ACT Web site at www.act.org before registering to take either test.

Your teenager does not have to be concerned that revealing his ADHD diagnosis will negatively affect his chances for admission. The Americans with Disabilities Act (ADA) bars discrimination against students with disabilities in the college application process, and admissions committees cannot legally discriminate against students with ADHD. Having a diagnosis of ADHD is much less important than a student's demonstrated ability to manage his schoolwork sufficiently to meet his school's academic standards. If your child's high school academic record has fallen short of his potential, a personal interview with a college admissions officer can provide a key format for discussing the reasons for his past difficulties and his plans for addressing them in the future. Meanwhile, an open attitude toward his academic strengths, weaknesses, and support needs may help him start his new life with a healthy attitude and an opportunity for greater success.

A student's acceptance into a college or university is an important landmark in the challenging process of transitioning from adolescence to independent adult life. To help smooth the way, some colleges offer summer programs prior to the beginning of the freshman year. These programs can be especially helpful for students with ADHD. Your teenager can further prepare for his freshman year by exploring his future college's library facilities, social opportunities, academic services, and other offerings on the Web; contacting his future roommate; talking with older students who can tell him more about the school; and talking with you and older siblings or family members about the challenges and joys he is likely to encounter the next school year.

YOUR COLLEGE STUDENT'S RIGHTS

Attention-deficit/hyperactivity disorder, when it substantially limits a major life activity (such as learning), is legally categorized as a disability under Section 504 of the Rehabilitation Act of 1973 and the ADA. Section 504, which applies to all colleges that receive federal funds—all public and most private colleges—prohibits discrimination against students with this type of disability and requires the colleges to provide the academic accommodations and services necessary to make courses, examinations, and activities accessible to these students.

The ADA provisions apply generally to public and private colleges, whether or not they receive federal funds. This act prohibits discrimination against otherwise qualified students with ADHD-related problems that substantially limit their learning, and requires those students to be provided with reasonable accommodations.

A student with ADHD may or may not choose to disclose his diagnosis when applying to college. If he does not want special accommodations during the SAT, ACT, or other testing, or during other aspects of the application process, he may decide to disclose his disability only after admission. Disclosure after admission, and registration with the college's special services office, is necessary to receive services and accommodations to meet his ADHD-related needs.

Adjusting to College Life

Social Life

From the day he moves into his college dormitory room, a student with ADHD will be confronted with an array of choices that can challenge any new college student. A most immediate concern may involve finding a place within the social network. In some cases, the effort to fit in at social gatherings and to form new friendships may lead to overindulging in alcohol or experimenting with illicit drugs. While this is the case for many students who then move on to a more balanced academic and social life, students with ADHD may be more likely to consider using marijuana or substances to ease their social discomfort, diminish general anxiety, or "numb" their ADHD-related symptoms. A family history of substance abuse, failure to use the college's academic and social support services, lack of confidence regarding the ability to succeed at school, or a treatment plan that has not prepared the student to manage his symptoms in healthy ways can all increase the risk for drug or alcohol abuse. (It is important to note that the use of stimulant medication as prescribed should not increase this risk and may, in fact, diminish it as it helps to decrease impulsive behavior.)

Before leaving for college, it can help to have a frank discussion about the high risk of early derailment through alcohol or drug abuse at college. Acknowledge the fact that growing up involves a great deal of experimentation, and that the temptation to go along with what others are doing will be high. At the same time, lack of sleep, poor diet, and constant partying (or a lack of social activity) can throw any student off balance, intensifying his anxiety or ADHD-related vulnerabilities so that he may be tempted to "self-medicate" with alcohol or drugs. Certainly, everyone makes mistakes during the difficult transition from adolescence to adulthood. The important thing for students is to maintain awareness of how well they are doing in all areas of functioning and to get help early if they find themselves in trouble. This is not the time to take a wait-and-see approach or to try to solve such problems on their own.

If a student will be taking medication or will need to make use of counseling services, it would be best to get a referral to an appropriate physician or psychologist (in or out of the student health service) before classes begin and to have the names, phone numbers, and e-mail addresses of key personnel in an appropriate place. If taking medication for his ADHD or other mental health conditions, your teen should bring a letter from his treating physician stating the diagnosis and treatment prescribed. He should transfer refills of these medications to someone on or near campus to facilitate the process of obtaining refills. If the need arises for treatment of other issues, the sooner he seeks help from a psychologist, counselor, residential advisor, or other university support person with whom he has familiarized himself when applying to the school, the sooner he can maintain control over his life and the fewer academic, social, and emotional setbacks he will experience.

Emotional Changes

Some students with ADHD welcome college life as a chance to "start over" in a place where no one knows that they have any special needs. However, if they neglect to attend to their study habits, carefully plan their study time, take medication, or attend counseling sessions, problems that they may have been able to overcome in high school through personal effort and a great deal of support from others may start to resurface or increase. This experience can be extremely demoralizing to a young adult just beginning an independent life. Again, the college students most able to avoid these setbacks are those who consciously balance their activities, study habits, sleep patterns, and social lives, and limit their drug and alcohol experimentation within the framework imposed by their ADHD-related needs and limitations. Obtaining support in this area, such as joining a college support group for students with ADHD, may help them with this type of healthy self-monitoring and encourage them in their efforts to integrate ADHD interventions into their adult life. However, for many students with ADHD this approach, although ideal, may not be enough and they may need to seek out support services to ensure success.

Academic Concerns

While social and emotional concerns may take center stage when a college freshman first arrives on campus, academic issues may soon follow and actually become more urgent. Ideally, a well-prepared student should arrive at college with a good idea of his academic strengths and weaknesses and some tested strategies for dealing with them. If he has already presented the documentation necessary to register with the college's special services office, he will have had the opportunity to learn about available services and accommodations and meet members of the services staff. Through early registration, online research, appointments with professors, and conversations with older students, a teenager with ADHD can also start to learn which professors and classes may be most appropriate within his range of choices. Some college students with ADHD have trouble advocating for themselves—asking a professor to allow them to take tests untimed or in a private room (if that has proved helpful in the past), getting permission to use a laptop computer or a human aide to take notes in class, requesting early registration, etc. Counselors in the special services office are usually available to help these students obtain the services or accommodations they need. It is important to request such modifications well ahead of time, rather than expecting a professor to agree to an accommodation on the day of the test or lecture.

College students with ADHD may find it useful to arrange for a "personal coach" (see Chapter 7) who serves as a daily monitor—someone who checks in briefly with him each day, asks him what his most important tasks are for that day and how he plans to accomplish them, and provides positive feedback and support for working toward his goals. While such coaches can help younger children with ADHD learn healthy habits of self-awareness and self-monitoring, they can be especially useful in helping college students bridge the gap between parental monitoring and full independence. Some special service offices at colleges and universities are beginning to provide such coaches, or references to off-campus coaching services, to students with ADHD. There is almost always an extra charge for this service. However, for a student who is struggling to stay on track as he adjusts to college life, a "coach" can make a critical difference.

Again, your child should be strongly encouraged and reminded to seek help early if he encounters problems with schoolwork, testing, or other academic issues. (See Chapter 11 for academic strategies that may improve his college performance.) In addition, academic and special supports available on campus are likely to include a freshman orientation, freshman experience course, residential advisor, freshman advisor, tutoring network, writing center, computer laboratory, counseling center, career counselor, health center, and fitness center. All of these services are paid for as part of his tuition, so they are readily available to him— and the sooner and more frequently he takes full advantage of them, the more on-track his college experience is likely to be.

Employment and the Workplace

While college life may be a challenge for any adolescent, life in the workplace can be just as formidable for a young adult with ADHD. Not only is he exposed to the same social and emotional pressures as his peers on college campuses, but he must also perform in a work environment that typically provides few or no supportive services and where no one may know he has ADHD. He may find it more stressful than he had expected to arrive at work exactly on time, manage paperwork or other detail-oriented work, attend frequent meetings, meet deadlines, and otherwise conform to what can often be a noisy, stressful and, in some cases, physically inactive environment. While teenagers with ADHD can often perform as well as their peers, adults with ADHD who are employed full-time tend to switch jobs more frequently and earn less money than their colleagues.

A young adult with ADHD will be more likely to start off on the right foot if he spends time during high school considering what types of jobs might best suit someone with his particular strengths and weaknesses and working on developing his time-management and self-care skills. Career counseling services are often available through the high school guidance office, and may be mandated under IDEA. Any job can be made more "ADHD-friendly" if the employee with ADHD knows how to alter his environment to better suit his needs and to advocate effectively for appropriate accommodations.

Coping With the Workplace

A teenager or young adult with ADHD who joins the workforce but finds a job too difficult should get some help in analyzing where the job-related challenges lie. Is he overwhelmed by paperwork? Does he get in trouble for arriving late on too many days? Does he put off tasks and thus fail to complete them? Does he forget his employer's instructions? Does he find it impossible to concentrate with all the noise around him? Is it hard for him to get along with coworkers or his boss?

Once he has identified his problem areas, he can brainstorm on his own or with coworkers, a job coach, a counselor or a psychologist, a family member, or members of his treatment team about ways to address them. He may decide to use a daily planner or computer software to manage daily tasks and appointments. A watch with alarms or a timer can help him keep track of work arrival time or deadlines, and any number of handheld devices can be used to record tasks to be accomplished. He may choose to carpool with a coworker to help him get to work on time, and to take regular, brief "exercise breaks" to work off excess energy. Many more such ideas are available on online support sites for adults with ADHD, such as www.add.org and www.chadd.org, and in books for adults with ADHD listed in the Resources section on page 311. Remember, there is no one-size-fits-all approach to these problems.

Asking Your Employer for Help

If these self-help techniques prove insufficient, and if a young adult feels comfortable disclosing that he has some functional issues related to ADHD, he should consider asking his employer about accommodations that might be provided that could help him work at his best level. Accommodations might include a less distracting office or workspace, a daily review each morning of work to be done, help with breaking complex jobs into smaller tasks, or even flex-time or a transfer from a heavily detail-oriented, time-pressured job to one that better matches his strengths. It may be difficult for him to work up the courage to ask for such help at first, but chances are that his employer will make at least some effort to cooperate. His problems at work may have puzzled or displeased his supervisor if she did not previously understand their cause, and she will probably appreciate and respect her employee's effort to improve his performance. As is the case in any aspect of his life, he is likely to meet with greater success on the job as he focuses on his strengths rather than his weaknesses. Adults with ADHD are often among the most creative, imaginative, energetic members of society. The more successfully he can understand and communicate to his employer his talents, strengths, and needs, the harder he or she may work to help him. It is important to remember, however, that ADHD symptoms are an explanation of why he is experiencing difficulty and not an excuse for them. The greater his understanding of how ADHD affects him and the better his self-esteem coming out of high school, the more likely he will feel empowered to effectively advocate for himself in a present or future job.

As was pointed out earlier in this chapter, an adolescent may be entitled to continue counseling services and assessment under an IDEA-mandated Individual Written Rehabilitation Plan. If this is not the case, however, he will need to be extra-vigilant regarding any ADHD-related concerns that are beginning to get out of hand, because routine accommodations are rarely provided by an employer. Make sure that your teenager has the names and phone numbers of physicians, job counselors, therapists, and other community resources who can help him with a variety of potential difficulties. The most helpful role as a parent may include providing nonjudgmental help or "reality checks" if he approaches you about these issues. Parents should remember that their role is to empower and not to enable or provide excuses for their adult child.

If he is offered a health insurance plan by his employer, he should review it along with his job-related benefits to learn in advance what counseling or other support services he can obtain. He may also consider the possible benefits of using a coach to help with some of these transitions from adolescence to adult life. Again, a thorough understanding of his ADHD-related strengths and weaknesses, coupled with a determination to monitor and manage his symptoms, is the best way for your growing adolescent to join the ranks of other young adults with ADHD who enjoy stimulating, fulfilling, and successful careers.

Health and Safety

A growing number of studies have shown that adults with ADHD may be at greater risk for health- and safety-related problems than their peers without ADHD. Their greater risk-taking behaviors and frequently erratic driving practices (inability to follow driving rules, inconsistent operation of vehicles) increase the chances of injuries. During adolescence and young adulthood, they may also have more unprotected sex with a greater number of partners than those without ADHD, and are therefore at greater risk for acquired immunodeficiency syndrome (AIDS) and other sexually transmitted infections.

It is important that your child be informed as early as the preteen and early teen years about these areas of increased risk. A healthy and proactive stance for a young adult with ADHD includes monitoring his risk-taking behaviors closely. In general, the more fully he understands that his health and safety are his own responsibility, and that monitoring his risk-taking behavior will always be an important part of his life, the better prepared he will be to meet these challenges. Switching to long-acting stimulant preparations or making sure symptoms are under control when driving or well into the evening hours may also help with critical decision-making and problem-solving skills affected by uncontrolled ADHD symptoms.

A Brief Look Forward: Adults With ADHD

If your child has experienced social rejection or problems with relationships during his early years, he may be concerned about how having the common problems associated with ADHD will affect his ability to enjoy a happy, fulfilling adult family life. In general, adults with ADHD may experience problems in the areas of long-term personal relationships and parenting. The ADHD-related symptoms, such as impulsiveness, inattention, and lack of organization, can disrupt family functioning—shifting most of the responsibility to other family members and thus generating a great deal of resentment and anger. Frequent job changes or the highs and lows of entrepreneurial life can also take their toll on family life.

Because ADHD tends to run in families, adults with the condition may find that some of their children share many of their own symptoms. Managing a child's ADHD-related behavior and consistently implementing approaches, such as behavior therapy techniques, can be particularly challenging for a parent who has ADHD. Hopefully, when your child reaches adulthood—having received careful evaluation, treatment, and monitoring throughout childhood and adolescence, and having been taught sound principles of behavior management as adults—he will find increasing success in family life and parenting.

As in academic life and on the job, a direct, forthright approach is often best when trying to minimize any effects of ADHD on personal relationships. Partners and children of an adult with ADHD are far more likely to accept and try to work around the lack of attention to their feelings and ideas if they understand where these concerns are coming from in the context of ADHD. Some common complaints of family members—that the person with ADHD is selfish, unperceptive, disorganized, forgetful, and takes too many risks—are all aspects of ADHD, not a personality defect or an indication that he does not love them. Efforts to communicate this fully to his partner and children—if necessary with the help of a counselor or family therapist—can go a long way toward putting his family life on the right track. Once the entire family understands how ADHD can affect behavior and influence personal interactions—once family members understand that the parent's or spouse's inattention or impulsiveness is not his "fault"—they can begin to identify problem areas in their daily lives and experiment with the best ways to address them. Typical relationship-enhancing approaches include

- **Understanding the need for structure.** Because adults with ADHD often lack structure in their inner lives, they may need more external structure if they are to function well. Partners of adults with ADHD often find that life goes more smoothly when family members routinely make lists of tasks to be done, maintain a family calendar to which everyone can refer, clarify which family member is responsible for which chores, and remind the person with ADHD, if necessary, of time constraints.
- **Breaking down tasks into manageable steps.** It may be possible to get through a mortgage application together or to plan a daughter's wedding without major setbacks—when partners agree to take it one step at a time.

- **Playing to each other's strengths.** If one partner is a more organized bill payer and the other can commit to driving the kids to their after-school activities, there is no reason why these tasks cannot be divided in the most acceptable and effective way. Taking on too much responsibility for daily chores is a major complaint of partners of adults with ADHD, so it is important to make sure that, even if the adult with ADHD is better off not being assigned deadline-oriented duties, he makes up for it by taking on other chores that are viewed by his partner as having an equal payoff value.

- **Learning how to communicate effectively.** Despite the best efforts by an adult with ADHD, his ADHD-related behaviors can still cause resentment in family members. Rather than expressing anger in non-productive ways, or risk intensifying the resentment by trying to talk about the issue with an inattentive partner, it may be better to agree ahead of time on a more effective way to communicate—over the phone, via e-mail, using a timer to ensure that each person has a chance to speak or, in times of major conflict, with the help of a family or couples therapist.

- **Maintaining realistic expectations.** Just as all adults have areas of strength and weakness, some adults with ADHD may never be able to handle the family's finances as well as their partner. If their partner is also unwilling or unable to take over responsibilities, it may be better to hire outside help than to blame a partner for his inadequacies.

- **Understanding that relationships are a 2-way street.** Couples and families need to take care that the entire burden to solve ADHD-related problems is not placed on the person with ADHD. Just as the adult with ADHD must work to manage his problems with organization or impulse control, his partner should try to support and facilitate his efforts. Mutual respect will help motivate all family members to continue doing their best.

- **Celebrating the joys of the partnership.** Adults with ADHD typically bring a great jolt of energy, spontaneity, inspiration, and excitement to marriage and family life. Couples should remember to take breaks from problem-solving to remember why they got together in the first place, and to appreciate what they have accomplished together and who they have become.

Specific techniques for addressing problems as they arise can be adapted from the earlier education and treatment experiences of the adult with ADHD, or both partners may be able to create new ones together and on their own. Ideas are also available on ADHD support Web sites and in books for adults with ADHD (see the Resources section on page 311).

Successful Arrival at Young Adulthood

Adults with ADHD are much more likely to enjoy successful and satisfying lives if they were properly prepared during childhood and adolescence to monitor and manage their symptoms on their own. Throughout this book, you have been encouraged as a parent to give your child the gift of self-empowerment—to include him in the process of understanding his symptoms; all decisions relating to his evaluation and treatment; discussions of the ways in which ADHD is affecting and may later affect his daily life; and planning for his future as a student, a family member, and a productive member of the adult world. By parenting to your child's strengths, continually building his knowledge base, taking care to applaud his efforts, and otherwise nurturing his self-esteem through childhood and adolescence, you have taught him to think of himself not as an "ADHD adult" but as an "adult who has ADHD."

Now as your teenager enters adulthood, armed with the knowledge, experience, and practiced ability to manage his ADHD-related symptoms, he will begin independent life in a stronger position than that of the generations who preceded him. Of course, every young adult with ADHD is different, and no individual outcome can be predicted. But by incorporating the guidelines presented in this book, and empowering him to use this information as you watch him proceed from childhood, through adolescence, to young adulthood, you will have helped your child take advantage of his unique strengths and take charge of his vulnerabilities as he begins his adult life.

Afterword

Direction for Future Research

The discussions in this book have been driven from the perspective of a rapidly growing body of research on all aspects of attention-deficit/hyperactivity disorder (ADHD). We all look forward to new advances and directions. Listed below are areas that will lead to even further advancement in our knowledge and success at helping to develop optimal outcomes.

- **Diagnosis.** The criteria for the diagnosis of ADHD are updated periodically by panels of experts. Researchers are currently studying the structure and functioning of the brain to better understand the characteristics of ADHD. In addition, genetic studies are being conducted that will help us understand the inherited nature of ADHD. These kinds of information may lead to advances in not only diagnostic process, but also contribute to a greater ability to target treatments for specific patients. Improved tools are needed to monitor the degree of the ADHD impairment.

- **Treatment.** The currently available treatments for ADHD are designed to manage the symptoms associated with this condition. While they are effective, they may have side effects that limit their use in some children, and they sometimes pose challenges over the long term. More research is needed that may lead to advances in medications that provide greater efficacy and limited side effects, and that better define the effectiveness and adverse effects of medications when they're used in combinations, such as a stimulant along with other agents. More information also needs to be collected on the use of medication in different age groups. In addition, there is a need to also continue to study and refine behavioral treatments and coaching interventions. Further research is also needed on how to enhance adherence to treatment since all the current treatments are symptomatic and frequently need to be sustained over long periods in order to benefit from the interventions.

- **Long-term effects of ADHD.** Because ADHD can continue into adulthood in many cases, researchers are conducting studies to find out more about the long-term outcomes and consequences of the disorder and its treatment. One goal is to be able to identify those children with ADHD who have a high risk of poorer long-term outcomes, so that new and more intensive treatments can be developed for them.

- **New measurement tools.** Researchers are also attempting to gain a better understanding of ADHD by developing new measurement tools that will help measure improvement as well as better ways to assess problems in different areas of functioning at different ages and stages of development.

Knowledge Is Power

Clearly, the better informed you and your child, as an adolescent and adult, are about new ADHD-related research and about ADHD across the life span, the more likely it is that he will benefit from these increases in our understanding of future treatment innovations. As your child makes the transition to adulthood, he should remain allied with professionals familiar with the latest studies regarding ADHD and coexisting conditions. He should also be familiar with the names and Web site addresses of the major national ADHD support and advocacy groups, such as Children and Adults with Attention Deficit Hyperactivity Disorder (CHADD) and Parent Advocacy Coalition for Educational Rights (PACER), and encouraged to check in with them and other reliable sources regularly for updates on recent ADHD-related research, as well as new legislation and sources of support. Thanks to CHADD, PACER, and similar organizations, children and adults with ADHD are much better served in the community than they were scant decades ago. As an adult, your growing child could benefit enormously from adding his own time and energy to these advocacy efforts.

Knowledge is power for children, adolescents, and adults with ADHD, and the gold standard to which you and your child should apply any new information is whether it will improve his functioning and enhance his self-esteem, relationships, school and job performance, happiness, and health. As a self-aware, self-monitoring, and self-confident individual, he will be well equipped to take advantage of the advances in ADHD-related knowledge, treatment, and practical support that are sure to come his way. As we stated in the introduction to this book, we remain optimistic that by using the approaches described here, and by updating your knowledge periodically from reliable sources, you will remain on the cutting edge of the most proven effective paths to an optimum outcome for your child.

Resources

This is not an all-inclusive resource list; however, the following suggestions will get you started in your search for information. Make sure that your pediatrician knows about your questions and concerns; share the information you've found. You and your pediatrician are partners in your child's health.

Please note: Listing of resources does not imply an endorsement by the American Academy of Pediatrics (AAP). The AAP is not responsible for the content of the resources. Phone numbers and Web site addresses are as current as possible, but may change at any time.

Associations

American Academy of Family Physicians (AAFP)
913/906-6000
800/274-2237
www.aafp.org
www.familydoctor.org

American Academy of Pediatrics (AAP)
847/434-4000
www.healthychildren.org (AAP parenting Web site)
www.aap.org

Attention Deficit Disorder Association (ADDA)
800/939-1019
www.add.org

Children and Adults with Attention Deficit/Hyperactivity Disorder (CHADD)
301/306-7070
800/233-4050
www.chadd.org

Learning Disabilities Association of America (LDA)

412/341-1515

www.ldanatl.org

National Dissemination Center for Children with Disabilities (NICHCY)

202/884-8200

800/695-0285

www.nichcy.org

National Tourette Syndrome Association, Inc. (TSA)

718/224-2999

www.tsa-usa.org

Parent Advocacy Coalition for Educational Rights (PACER)

952/838-9000

www.pacer.org

Government Organizations

Centers for Disease Control and Prevention (CDC)

800/CDC-INFO

www.cdc.gov (Search Health and Safety Topics for ADHD)

www.cdc.gov/ncbddd/adhd/

National Institute of Mental Health (NIMH)

866/615-6464

www.nimh.nih.gov (Search Mental Health Topics for ADHD)

http://www.nimh.nih.gov/health/topics/attention-deficit-hyperactivity-disorder-adhd/index.shtml

United States Department of Education

800/USA-LEARN

www.ed.gov

http://www2.ed.gov/nclb/landing.jhtml (For information on the Elementary and Secondary Education Act)

www.eric.ed.gov (Education Resources Information Center [ERIC])

Other ADHD Resources Available on the Internet

About Our Kids (NYU Child Study Center)

www.aboutourkids.org (Search A to Z Disorder Guide for ADHD)

ADDvance Answers to Your Questions about ADD (ADHD)

www.addvance.com

Center for Children and Families

http://ccf.buffalo.edu

Developmental and Behavioral Pediatrics Online

www.dbpeds.org (Professional site with handouts of interest to parents)

National Resource Center on ADHD

www.help4adhd.org (A program of CHADD)

Teaching LD: Information & Resources for Teaching Students with Learning Disabilities

www.dldcec.org

Books for Parents, Teachers, and College Students

General

Barkley RA. *Taking Charge of ADHD: The Complete, Authoritative Guide for Parents.* 2nd ed. New York, NY: Guilford Press; 2000

Fowler M. *Maybe You Know My Teen: A Parent's Guide to Helping Your Adolescent With Attention Deficit/Hyperactivity Disorder.* New York, NY: Broadway Books; 2001

Hallowell EM, Jensen PS. *Superparenting for ADD: An Innovative Approach to Raising Your Distracted Child.* New York, NY: Ballantine Books; 2010

Hallowell EM, Ratey JJ. *Delivered from Distraction: Getting the Most out of Life with Attention Deficit Disorder.* New York, NY: Ballantine Books; 2005

Jensen PS. *Making the System Work for Your Child With ADHD.* New York, NY: Guilford Press, 2004

Nadeau KG. *ADD in the Workplace: Choices, Changes, and Challenges.* Philadelphia, PA: Routledge; 1997

Nadeau KG. *Survival Guide for College Students with ADD or LD.* Washington, DC: Magination Press; 1994

Nadeau KG. *Adventures in Fast Forward: Life, Love and Work for the ADD Adult.* Philadelphia, PA: Rutledge; 1996

Nadeau KG, Littman EB, Quinn PO. *Understanding Girls with AD/HD.* Silver Spring, MD: Advantage Books; 2000

Parker HC. *The ADD Hyperactivity Workbook for Parents, Teachers and Kids.** Plantation, FL: Specialty Press; 1999

Quinn PO, ed. *ADD and the College Student: A Guide for High School and College Students with Attention Deficit Disorder.* Washington, DC: Magination Press; 2001

Robin AL. *ADHD in Adolescents: Diagnosis and Treatment.* New York, NY: Guildford Press; 1999

Wilens TE. *Straight Talk about Psychiatric Medications for Kids.* 3rd ed. New York, NY: Guilford Press; 2008

*Available in Spanish

ADHD and School

Anderson W, Chitwood S, Hayden D. *Negotiating the Special Education Maze.* 4th ed. Bethesda, MD: Woodbine House; 2008

Dawson P, Guare R. *Smart but Scattered: The Revolutionary "Executive Skills" Approach to Helping Kids Reach Their Potential.* New York, NY: Guilford Press; 2009

Power TJ, Karustis JL, Habboushe DF. *Homework Success for Children with ADHD: A Family-School Intervention Program.* New York, NY: Guilford Press; 2001

Reif SF. *How to Reach and Teach ADD/ADHD Students: Practical Techniques, Strategies, and Interventions.* 2nd ed. San Francisco, CA: Jossey-Bass; 2005

Smith C, Strick L. *Learning Disabilities from A to Z: A Complete Guide to Learning Disabilities from Preschool to Adolescence.* Rev ed. New York, NY: Free Press; 2010

Zentall SS. *ADHD and Education: Foundations, Characteristics, Methods and Collaboration.* Upper Saddle River, NJ: Prentice Hall; 2006

Behavior Management and Social Skills

Barkley RA, Benton CM. *Your Defiant Child: Eight Steps to Better Behavior.* New York, NY: Guilford Press; 1998

Christophersen ER, Mortweet SL. *Parenting That Works: Building Skills That Last a Lifetime.* Washington, DC: American Psychological Association; 2003

Greene RW. *The Explosive Child: A New Approach for Understanding and Parenting Easily Frustrated, Chronically Inflexible Children.* 4th ed. New York, NY: Harper Paperbacks; 2010

Heininger JE, Weiss SK. *From Chaos to Calm: Effective Parenting of Challenging Children with ADHD and other Behavioral Problems.* New York, NY: Perigree Books; 2001

Coexisting Conditions

Koplewicz HS. *More Than Moody: Recognizing and Treating Adolescent Depression.* New York, NY: Penguin Group; 2002

Marsh TL. *Children with Tourette Syndrome: A Parent's Guide.* Bethesda, MD: Woodbine House; 2007

National Institute of Mental Health. *Bipolar Disorder in Children and Teens: A Parent's Guide.* NIH Publication No. 08-6380. Bethesda, MD: National Institute of Mental Health

Ozonoff S, Dawson G. *A Parent's Guide to Asperger Syndrome and High-Functioning Autism: How to Meet the Challenges and Help Your Child Thrive.* New York, NY: Guilford Press; 2002

Books for Children and Adolescents With ADHD

Younger Children

Corman C, Trevino E. *Eukee the Jumpy Jumpy Elephant.* Plantation, FL: Specialty Press; 1996
An entertaining way for your young child to learn about ADHD.

Galvin M. *Otto Learns About His Medicine: A Story About Medication for Children with ADHD.* 3rd ed. Washington, DC: Magination Press; 2001
An illustrated introduction for children about taking medication for ADHD.

Gordon M. *Jumpin' Johnny Get Back to Work! A Child's Guide to ADHD/Hyperactivity.* * **
DeWitt, NY: Gordon Systems; 1991

Roberts B. *Phoebe Flower's Adventures: That's What Kids Are For.* Bethesda, MD: Advantage Books; 1998
Series for children starring a young girl with ADHD—one of the few stories that features a girl.

*Available in Spanish
** Available as a video

Older Children

Gehret J. *Teaching with I'm Somebody Too.* Fairport, NY: Verbal Images Press; 1996
Novel told by the sister of a boy with ADD. Explains ADD and how it affects a family.

Gordon M. *I Would If I Could: A Teenager's Guide to ADHD/Hyperactivity.* DeWitt, NY: Gordon Systems; 1992
Acknowledges the unique experience of a child with ADHD, offering the reader a humorous, empathetic forum for exploring his own feelings.

Gordon M. *My Brother's a World Class Pain.* DeWitt, NY: Gordon System; 1992
A book for siblings of children with ADHD.

Ingersoll BD. *Distant Drums, Different Drummers: A Guide for Young People with ADHD.* Bethesda, MD: Cape Publicationss; 1995
Stresses a positive perspective and the value of individual differences.

Quinn P, Stern J. *Putting On the Brakes: Young People's Guide to Understanding Attention Deficit Hyperactivity Disorder.* Washington, DC: Magination Press; 2001

A guide to ADHD written about entering adolescence.

Adolescents

Nadeau KG. *Help4ADD@High School.* Bethesda, MD: Advantage Press; 1998

A book written in an entertaining Web site format, providing useful information on how students can help themselves in school.

Quinn PO. *Adolescents and ADD: Gaining the Advantage.* Washington, DC: Magination Press; 1995

Ziegler Dendy CA, Ziegler A. *A Bird's Eye View of Life with ADD and ADHD: Advice From Young Survivors.* 2nd ed. Cedar Bluff, AL: Cherish the Children; 2007

Magazines and Newsletters

ADDitude

888/762-8475

www.additudemag.com

A commercially produced magazine for families and adults living with ADHD and learning disabilities.

ATTENTION!

800/233-4050

www.chadd.org

A magazine offering support and information for people affected by ADHD. Available with membership to CHADD.

Healthy Children

www.aap.org/healthychildren

Magazine of the American Academy of Pediatrics featuring a wide range of health topics, including developmental and behavioral issues.

ADHD Book and Video Resources

A.D.D. WareHouse

800/233-9273

www.addwarehouse.com

Childswork/Childsplay

800/962-1141

www.childswork.com

Appendix

Vanderbilt Assessment Scales

D3	**NICHQ Vanderbilt Assessment Scale—PARENT Informant**

Today's Date: _____ Child's Name: _____ Date of Birth: _____

Parent's Name: _____ Parent's Phone Number: _____

Directions: Each rating should be considered in the context of what is appropriate for the age of your child.
When completing this form, please think about your child's behaviors in the past **6 months.**

Is this evaluation based on a time when the child ☐ was on medication   ☐ was not on medication   ☐ not sure?

Symptoms	Never	Occasionally	Often	Very Often
1. Does not pay attention to details or makes careless mistakes with, for example, homework	0	1	2	3
2. Has difficulty keeping attention to what needs to be done	0	1	2	3
3. Does not seem to listen when spoken to directly	0	1	2	3
4. Does not follow through when given directions and fails to finish activities (not due to refusal or failure to understand)	0	1	2	3
5. Has difficulty organizing tasks and activities	0	1	2	3
6. Avoids, dislikes, or does not want to start tasks that require ongoing mental effort	0	1	2	3
7. Loses things necessary for tasks or activities (toys, assignments, pencils, or books)	0	1	2	3
8. Is easily distracted by noises or other stimuli	0	1	2	3
9. Is forgetful in daily activities	0	1	2	3
10. Fidgets with hands or feet or squirms in seat	0	1	2	3
11. Leaves seat when remaining seated is expected	0	1	2	3
12. Runs about or climbs too much when remaining seated is expected	0	1	2	3
13. Has difficulty playing or beginning quiet play activities	0	1	2	3
14. Is "on the go" or often acts as if "driven by a motor"	0	1	2	3
15. Talks too much	0	1	2	3
16. Blurts out answers before questions have been completed	0	1	2	3
17. Has difficulty waiting his or her turn	0	1	2	3
18. Interrupts or intrudes in on others' conversations and/or activities	0	1	2	3
19. Argues with adults	0	1	2	3
20. Loses temper	0	1	2	3
21. Actively defies or refuses to go along with adults' requests or rules	0	1	2	3
22. Deliberately annoys people	0	1	2	3
23. Blames others for his or her mistakes or misbehaviors	0	1	2	3
24. Is touchy or easily annoyed by others	0	1	2	3
25. Is angry or resentful	0	1	2	3
26. Is spiteful and wants to get even	0	1	2	3
27. Bullies, threatens, or intimidates others	0	1	2	3
28. Starts physical fights	0	1	2	3
29. Lies to get out of trouble or to avoid obligations (ie, "cons" others)	0	1	2	3
30. Is truant from school (skips school) without permission	0	1	2	3
31. Is physically cruel to people	0	1	2	3
32. Has stolen things that have value	0	1	2	3

Copyright © 2005 American Academy of Pediatrics, University of North Carolina at Chapel Hill for its North Carolina Center for Children's Healthcare Improvement, and National Initiative for Children's Healthcare Quality

Adapted from the Vanderbilt Rating Scales developed by Mark L. Wolraich, MD.

Revised - 1102
11-19/rep1210

American Academy of Pediatrics
DEDICATED TO THE HEALTH OF ALL CHILDREN™

NICHQ
National Initiative for Children's Healthcare Quality

HE0350

D3	NICHQ Vanderbilt Assessment Scale—PARENT Informant, continued

Today's Date: _____ Child's Name: _____ Date of Birth: _____

Parent's Name: _____ Parent's Phone Number: _____

Symptoms (continued)	Never	Occasionally	Often	Very Often
33. Deliberately destroys others' property	0	1	2	3
34. Has used a weapon that can cause serious harm (bat, knife, brick, gun)	0	1	2	3
35. Is physically cruel to animals	0	1	2	3
36. Has deliberately set fires to cause damage	0	1	2	3
37. Has broken into someone else's home, business, or car	0	1	2	3
38. Has stayed out at night without permission	0	1	2	3
39. Has run away from home overnight	0	1	2	3
40. Has forced someone into sexual activity	0	1	2	3
41. Is fearful, anxious, or worried	0	1	2	3
42. Is afraid to try new things for fear of making mistakes	0	1	2	3
43. Feels worthless or inferior	0	1	2	3
44. Blames self for problems, feels guilty	0	1	2	3
45. Feels lonely, unwanted, or unloved; complains that "no one loves him or her"	0	1	2	3
46. Is sad, unhappy, or depressed	0	1	2	3
47. Is self-conscious or easily embarrassed	0	1	2	3

Performance	Excellent	Above Average	Average	Somewhat of a Problem	Problematic
48. Overall school performance	1	2	3	4	5
49. Reading	1	2	3	4	5
50. Writing	1	2	3	4	5
51. Mathematics	1	2	3	4	5
52. Relationship with parents	1	2	3	4	5
53. Relationship with siblings	1	2	3	4	5
54. Relationship with peers	1	2	3	4	5
55. Participation in organized activities (eg, teams)	1	2	3	4	5

Comments:

For Office Use Only

Total number of questions scored 2 or 3 in questions 1–9: _____

Total number of questions scored 2 or 3 in questions 10–18: _____

Total Symptom Score for questions 1–18:_____

Total number of questions scored 2 or 3 in questions 19–26: _____

Total number of questions scored 2 or 3 in questions 27–40: _____

Total number of questions scored 2 or 3 in questions 41–47: _____

Total number of questions scored 4 or 5 in questions 48–55: _____

Average Performance Score:_____

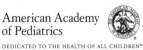

American Academy of Pediatrics

DEDICATED TO THE HEALTH OF ALL CHILDREN™

NICHQ

National Initiative for Children's Healthcare Quality

D4	**NICHQ Vanderbilt Assessment Scale—TEACHER Informant**

Teacher's Name: _____ Class Time: _____ Class Name/Period: _____

Today's Date: _____ Child's Name: _____ Grade Level: _____

Directions: Each rating should be considered in the context of what is appropriate for the age of the child you are rating and should reflect that child's behavior since the beginning of the school year. Please indicate the number of weeks or months you have been able to evaluate the behaviors: _____.

Is this evaluation based on a time when the child ☐ was on medication ☐ was not on medication ☐ not sure?

Symptoms	Never	Occasionally	Often	Very Often
1. Fails to give attention to details or makes careless mistakes in schoolwork	0	1	2	3
2. Has difficulty sustaining attention to tasks or activities	0	1	2	3
3. Does not seem to listen when spoken to directly	0	1	2	3
4. Does not follow through on instructions and fails to finish schoolwork (not due to oppositional behavior or failure to understand)	0	1	2	3
5. Has difficulty organizing tasks and activities	0	1	2	3
6. Avoids, dislikes, or is reluctant to engage in tasks that require sustained mental effort	0	1	2	3
7. Loses things necessary for tasks or activities (school assignments, pencils, or books)	0	1	2	3
8. Is easily distracted by extraneous stimuli	0	1	2	3
9. Is forgetful in daily activities	0	1	2	3
10. Fidgets with hands or feet or squirms in seat	0	1	2	3
11. Leaves seat in classroom or in other situations in which remaining seated is expected	0	1	2	3
12. Runs about or climbs excessively in situations in which remaining seated is expected	0	1	2	3
13. Has difficulty playing or engaging in leisure activities quietly	0	1	2	3
14. Is "on the go" or often acts as if "driven by a motor"	0	1	2	3
15. Talks excessively	0	1	2	3
16. Blurts out answers before questions have been completed	0	1	2	3
17. Has difficulty waiting in line	0	1	2	3
18. Interrupts or intrudes on others (eg, butts into conversations/games)	0	1	2	3
19. Loses temper	0	1	2	3
20. Actively defies or refuses to comply with adults' requests or rules	0	1	2	3
21. Is angry or resentful	0	1	2	3
22. Is spiteful and vindictive	0	1	2	3
23. Bullies, threatens, or intimidates others	0	1	2	3
24. Initiates physical fights	0	1	2	3
25. Lies to obtain goods for favors or to avoid obligations (eg, "cons" others)	0	1	2	3
26. Is physically cruel to people	0	1	2	3
27. Has stolen items of nontrivial value	0	1	2	3
28. Deliberately destroys others' property	0	1	2	3
29. Is fearful, anxious, or worried	0	1	2	3
30. Is self-conscious or easily embarrassed	0	1	2	3
31. Is afraid to try new things for fear of making mistakes	0	1	2	3

Copyright © 2005 American Academy of Pediatrics, University of North Carolina at Chapel Hill for its North Carolina Center for Children's Healthcare Improvement, and National Initiative for Children's Healthcare Quality

Adapted from the Vanderbilt Rating Scales developed by Mark L. Wolraich, MD.

Revised - 0303
11-20/rep0210

HE0351

American Academy of Pediatrics

DEDICATED TO THE HEALTH OF ALL CHILDREN™

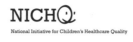

NICHQ

National Initiative for Children's Healthcare Quality

D4   **NICHQ Vanderbilt Assessment Scale—TEACHER Informant, continued**

Teacher's Name: _____ Class Time: _____ Class Name/Period: _____

Today's Date: _____ Child's Name: _____ Grade Level: _____

Symptoms (continued)	Never	Occasionally	Often	Very Often
32. Feels worthless or inferior	0	1	2	3
33. Blames self for problems; feels guilty	0	1	2	3
34. Feels lonely, unwanted, or unloved; complains that "no one loves him or her"	0	1	2	3
35. Is sad, unhappy, or depressed	0	1	2	3

Performance *Academic Performance*	Excellent	Above Average	Average	Somewhat of a Problem	Problematic
36. Reading	1	2	3	4	5
37. Mathematics	1	2	3	4	5
38. Written expression	1	2	3	4	5

Classroom Behavioral Performance	Excellent	Above Average	Average	Somewhat of a Problem	Problematic
39. Relationship with peers	1	2	3	4	5
40. Following directions	1	2	3	4	5
41. Disrupting class	1	2	3	4	5
42. Assignment completion	1	2	3	4	5
43. Organizational skills	1	2	3	4	5

Comments:

Please return this form to: _____

Mailing address: _____

_____

Fax number: _____

For Office Use Only

Total number of questions scored 2 or 3 in questions 1–9: _____

Total number of questions scored 2 or 3 in questions 10–18: _____

Total Symptom Score for questions 1–18: _____

Total number of questions scored 2 or 3 in questions 19–28: _____

Total number of questions scored 2 or 3 in questions 29–35: _____

Total number of questions scored 4 or 5 in questions 36–43: _____

Average Performance Score: _____

American Academy
of Pediatrics
DEDICATED TO THE HEALTH OF ALL CHILDREN™

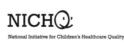

NICHQ
National Initiative for Children's Healthcare Quality

Index

A

O

Obsessive-compulsive disorder (OCD), 215–217
OCD. *See* Obsessive-compulsive disorder (OCD)
ODD. *See* Oppositional defiant disorder (ODD)
Open-plan design, 147
Oppositional defiant disorder (ODD), 200. *See also* Disruptive behavior disorders
Optometric training, 246–247
Organization, 177
Organizational and study skills, 164
Orthomolecular psychiatry, 239
Osmond, Humphry, 238, 239
"Other health impaired," 152
Outgrowing the condition, 7

P

PACER. *See* Parent Advocacy Coalition for Educational Rights (PACER)
Parent. *See also* Home life
adolescents, and, 277–283
anxiety, and, 208
care manager, as, 43–44, 97
child's advocate, as, 104
continuing responsibilities, 57
depression, and, 213–215
homework tips, 168–169
keep up-to-date, 105
narrating your behavior, 102, 119
ODD/CD, and, 204
organize your family life, 88
record keeping, 97–98
regroup, 88
supportive presence, as, 103
take care of yourself, 100, 136
talking to child about medication, 79–82
what to tell others, 36–37
Parent Advocacy Coalition for Educational Rights (PACER), 189, 308, 312
Parent taxi, 277
Parent training. See Behavior therapy
Parent's story
early start to treatment, 72
feeling involved, 260
Keller, Emma, 2
missed dues/lost opportunities, 14, 61
parenting approaches, 110
Scott, Andrew, 1

support system, 104
team effort, 55
Paroxetine, 78, 213
Passion flower, 241
Paul Wellstone and Pete Domenici Mental Health Parity and Addiction Equity Act, 193
Pauling, Linus, 239
Paxil, 78, 213
Pediatrician
coexisting conditions, 31, 198–199
dosage, 68
evaluation process, 20, 22
follow-up visits, 53, 54
functional impairment, 28
monitoring the results, 73
questions about school, 20
reports, 22
review findings with parent, 31
teacher, and, 170
Peer relationships, 101–103
Peer review, 236
Personal coach/trainer, 171–172
Personal stories. *See* Parent's story
Pervasive developmental disorders (PPDs), 196, 227
Phobia, 203
Phonologic awareness, 219, 224
Phonologic disorder, 224
Phosphatylserine, 241
Placebo, 235
Play therapy, 115, 135, 136
Positive reinforcement, 122, 124–127
Post-secondary education. *See* College
PPDs. *See* Pervasive developmental disorders (PPDs)
Praise, 90, 119, 121, 124
spoiling of, 122
techniques for, 122–123
Pre-referral interventions, 152
Predominantly hyperactive/impulsive-type attention-deficit/hyperactivity disorder, 19
Predominantly inattentive-type attention-deficit/hyperactivity disorder, 18
Preschool children
evaluation and diagnosis, 26, 27, 28–29
hyperactivity, 27
impulsivity, 27
inattention, 26
stimulant medications, 72–73